D0190804

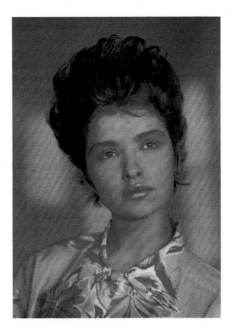

THE HAMLYN BASIC GUIDE TO

Hair care & styling

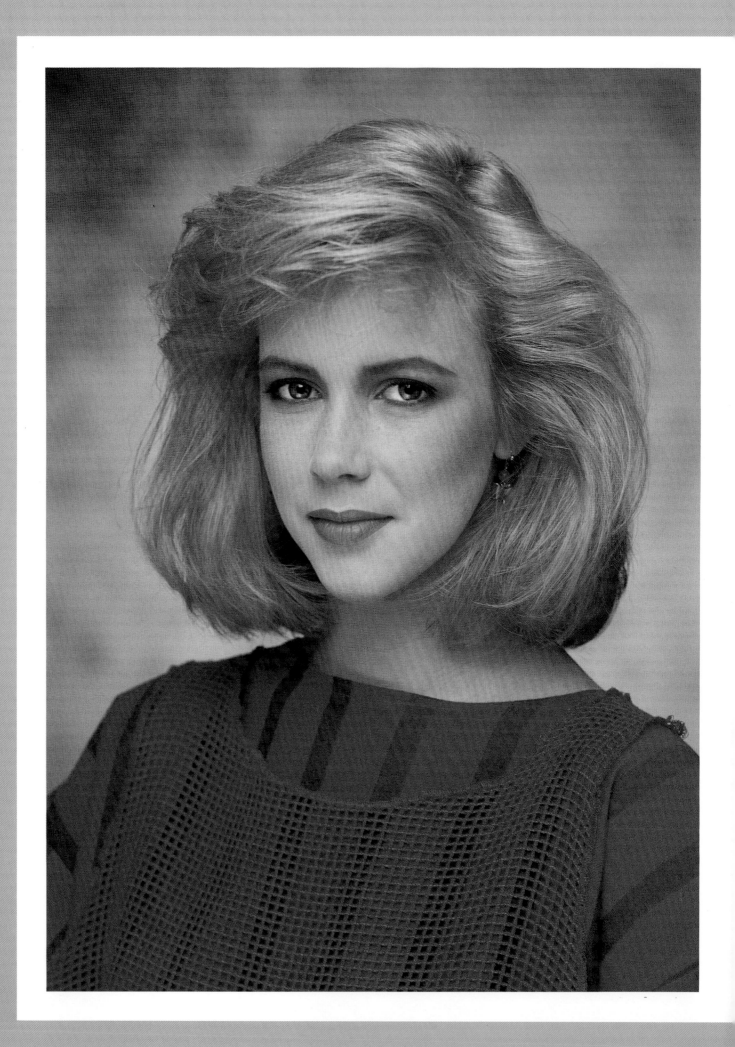

THE HAMLYN BASIC GUIDE TO

Hair care & styling

Jan Kettle

HAMLYN

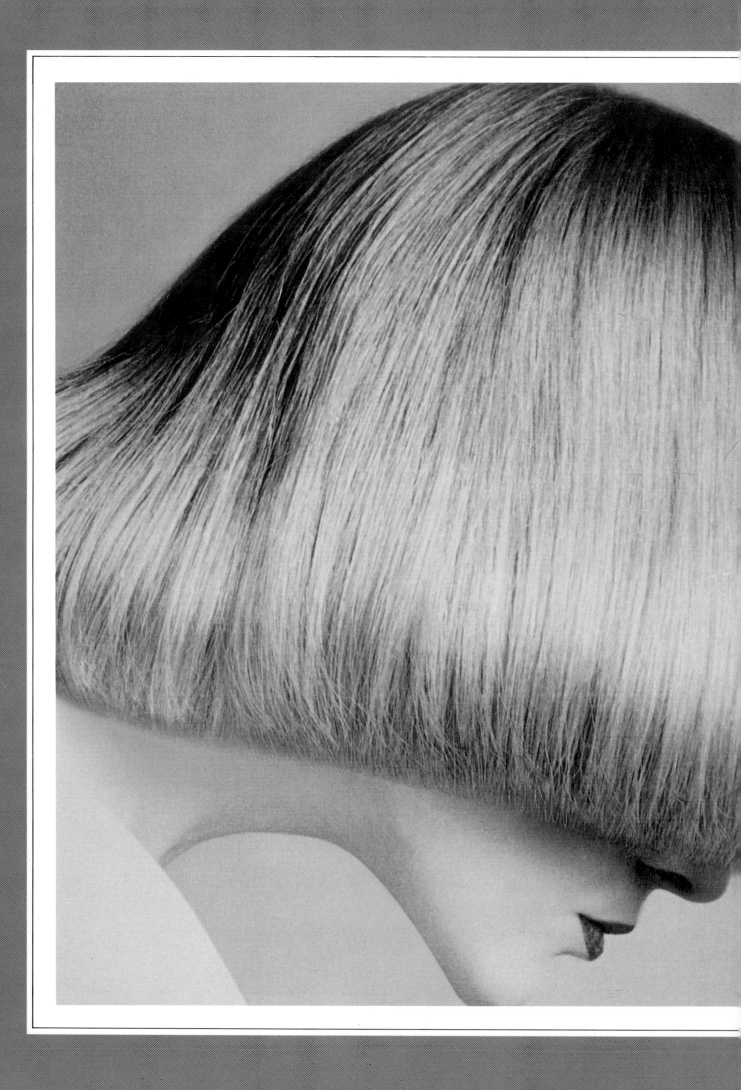

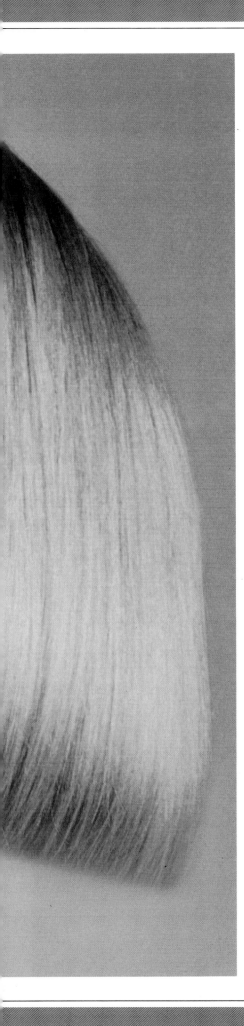

Contents

First published in 1986 by
Hamlyn Publishing,
Bridge House, London Road,
Twickenham, Middlesex

Copyright © Hamlyn Publishing 1986, a division of The Hamlyn
Publishing Group Limited

ISBN 0 600 50105 1

Printed in Spain by Cayfosa. Barcelona
Dep. Leg. B - 2573 - 1986

Cover photographs:
Background by Chris Crofton
Front inset by Al MacDonald, courtesy of Alberto TRESemme/Indola
Back inset courtesy of Schwarzkopf

Half title page: Photograph courtesy of L'Oréal
Title page: Photograph courtesy of Schwarzkopf
Contents page: Photograph courtesy of Crimpers of London

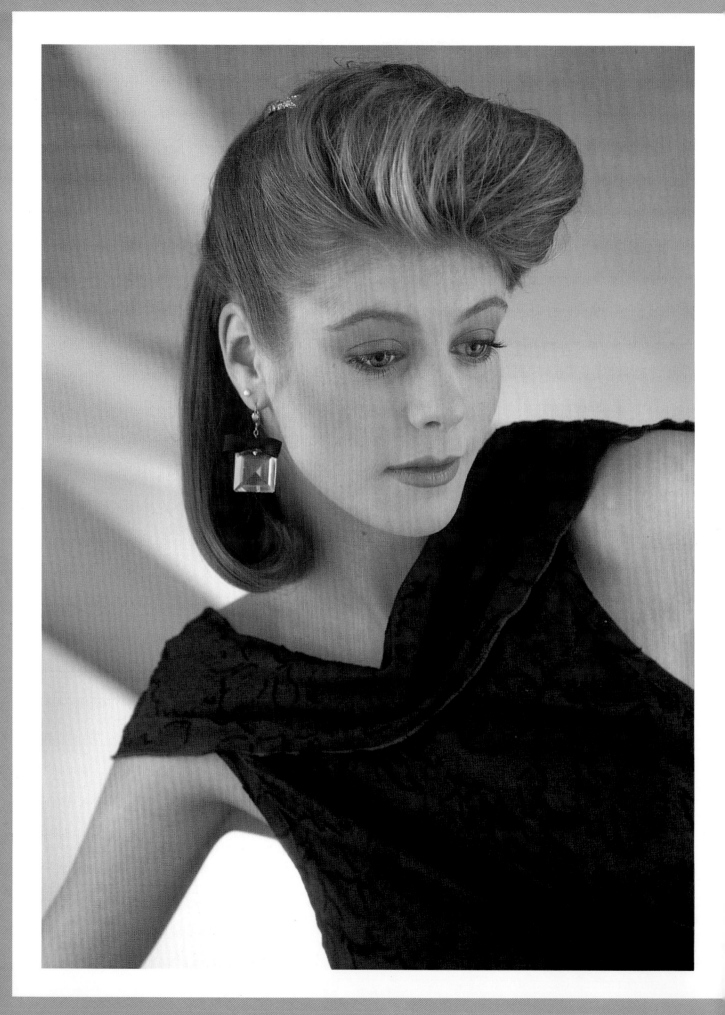

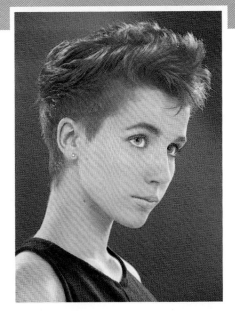

Introduction

My introduction to the world of hairdressing came three years ago. Up until then. I had considered that I was doing all the right things and was being as kind to my hair as anyone could be. It did not take me long to realize how brutally I had been treating it, with constant chemical treatments and daily subjection to heat, and how lightly I had been let off with mildly damaged hair which was still redeemable. Subsequently my thoughts on hair were totally restructured. During more than two years with *Hair & Beauty* magazine I worked closely with hairdressers and, in addition to realizing how warm and helpful most of them are, I also witnessed a revolution in hair fashion.

Hairdressers in the UK have a reputation for being just about the best there are. They are in constant demand at shows and seminars worldwide, and their hair pictures are frequently published in magazines in all the fashion-conscious countries. Their acclaim has not just been won by virtue of artistic talent. The economic recession has meant that over the past few years hairdressers have had to sharpen their philosophies as well as their scissors. They have smartened up not only their salons but the way in which they think about their clients. As a result, today's best hairdressers genuinely care about what kind of people their clients are, what suits them and, most of all, what they want. In many cases a hairdresser's knowledge of his customers is so well tuned that he almost deserves a degree in psychology.

Yet, as a beauty and hair journalist, I am still constantly barraged with the criticism that hairdressers never get it right. However, the craft has developed into a two-way communication between client and hairdresser, and it's as important for you, the customer, to be honest about the kind of person you are and about what you want, as it is for your stylist to tell you what he feels might or might not suit you. Finding the right person and developing that relationship is as important with your hairdresser as it is with your partner for life, if you are ever going to be happy with your hair.

In this book I hope not only to shed some light on this mysterious fibre on our heads which makes or breaks our appearance, but to help you overcome the obstacles and eventually find the hairdresser who is right for you.

In no other place and at no other time than in Britain today has hairdressing been better. Your time in a salon should be an enjoyable one and it should endow you with a head of hair which is an antidote to life's little setbacks. With the help of this book, those of you who have ever regarded your crowning glory as the bane of your life should never do so again.

Hair fashion knows no rules.
Opposite: A classic, side-swept style courtesy of *Hair & Beauty* magazine.
Above: A boyish, tousled style from the Stevie Buckle Hair Salon, London.

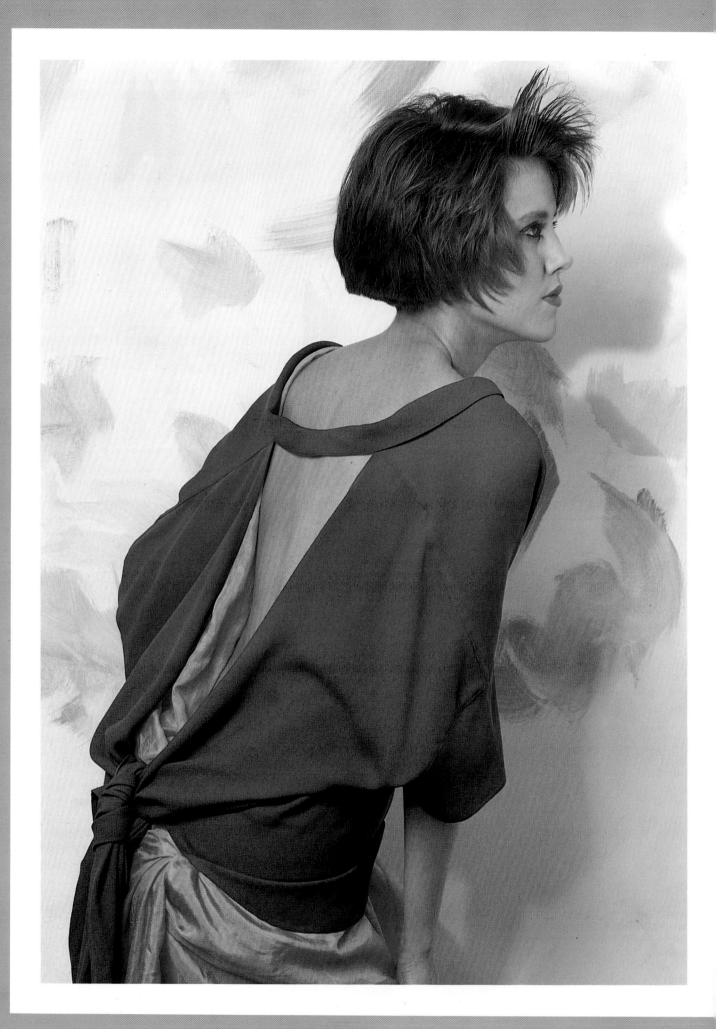

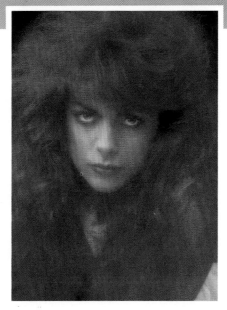

Understanding your hair

Of all the outfits which we possess to enhance our looks, hair is the one we never take off. A good well-conditioned style can turn heads in the street and boost our self-confidence in exactly the same way as an expensive outfit. Yet it is the one aspect of our personal appearance that we take for granted above all others.

From childhood to old age we abuse our hair through carelessness or sheer ignorance. We tug it back into damaging elastic bands, rip the ends apart by grooming incorrectly and even pull it out by the roots! We pursue this path of destruction by using harmful brushes and combs, by shampooing inadequately and by subjecting our hair to the intense rays of the sun. We complete the process by continual use of chemicals, sometimes applied inexpertly by amateurs, until our former crowning glory breaks beyond the point of no return. Then we panic.

Opposite: A short bob with a classic, romantic appeal from the Molton Brown Salon in London. **Above:** An equally classic style on more traditional long hair, which has first been gelled and pinned up in sections before being pulled down and brushed for a soft effect (by the Crimpers Salons, London).

Ignorance of this vital aspect of our looks has been with us since time immemorial. Hair has sometimes been revered, often abused. The early Egyptians shaved their heads, partly for religious reasons but also as a way of coping with the hot climate and of keeping their heads free from vermin. They progressed from one extreme to another as more elaborate styles became the fashion, and eventually wigs were worn by both men and women. Ancient Greeks preferred more natural hair and women spent great sums of money on oils and perfumes for it. According to legend, the ancient Romans believed that too-frequent washing disturbed the spirit guarding the head – so women were permitted to wash their hair only as often as once a year!

However, it was during supposedly more civilized times that hair care really suffered at the fickle fingers of fashion. During the 18th century incredibly extravagant creations would be filled with cotton wool and moulded together. Because they would not be disturbed for weeks, nests of mice were sometimes found to have taken up residence!

Hair make-up

The hair and scalp are two such delicately linked and intricate subjects that one can understand why countless generations before us have preferred to remain in blissful ignorance of them. But, whether we like it or not, first impressions are formed on appearances and our hair is very often the first part of us to be noticed. Hair care plays a more prominent part in beauty routines now than ever before, yet it is still often neglected – simply because it is least understood. So what exactly is hair and how is it formed?

Hair is a slender, thread-like extension of the skin. There are between 80,000 and 150,000 hairs on the human head at any one time, depending on gender and hair colour. A natural blonde tends to have more hairs on the scalp than a redhead and women tend to have more than men. But all of these hairs, or at least those which are visible to the human eye, are dead; it is from a root deep beneath the scalp, or the papilla, that life goes on.

The scalp is made up of three layers; the epidermis, the dermis and the hypodermis. The epidermis, more commonly known as the skin, has a life cycle of between five and six weeks and is itself divided up into layers. The epidermis is fed by the dermis, which is the home of the hair follicle where the hair actually begins its life. It is at the base of the follicle where the papilla is found and where the hair cells are produced. Living cells need nutrition and our hair cells draw theirs from blood vessels, which also feed the sebaceous glands with sulphur. The sebaceous glands are attached to the hair follicle and produce sebum which lubricates the hair shaft and scalp. For some people sebum is automatically associated with oiliness and is a dirty word, but it is vital to the well-being of our hair because it seals in essential moisture which protects it from dangerous elements such as the sun,

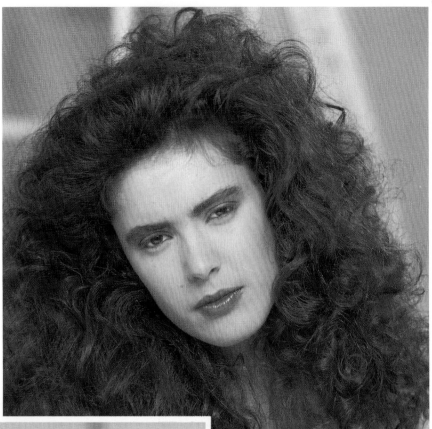

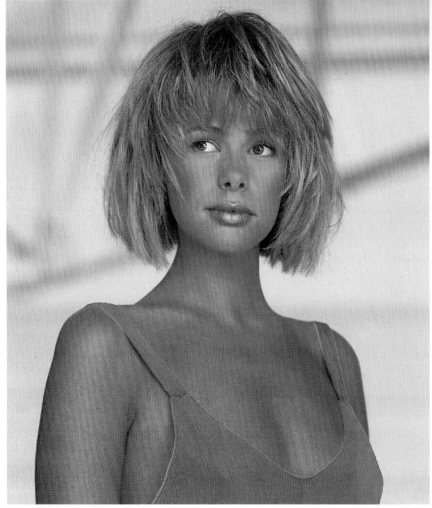

Above: Redheads often seem to have the most abundant hair type, but in fact they have the fewest number of hairs on the head (hair by Bastian for Alberto TRESemme/Indola). **Left:** Blondes have the greatest number of hairs, but these are much finer than red hair (courtesy of L'Oréal)

wind and weather; it also contains a natural antiseptic which helps fight infection. Sulphur supplied by the blood vessels controls the flow of sebum. The dermis also contains the nerves and nerve cells which are sensitive to touch, heat and movement. The third layer of the scalp, the hypodermis, is situated at the base of the dermis and is made up of fatty tissue which produces the fatty acids present in sebum.

The hair itself, or hair shaft, is also divided into three layers: the cuticle, cortex and medulla. The cuticle is the outer layer of the hair and its protective coating.

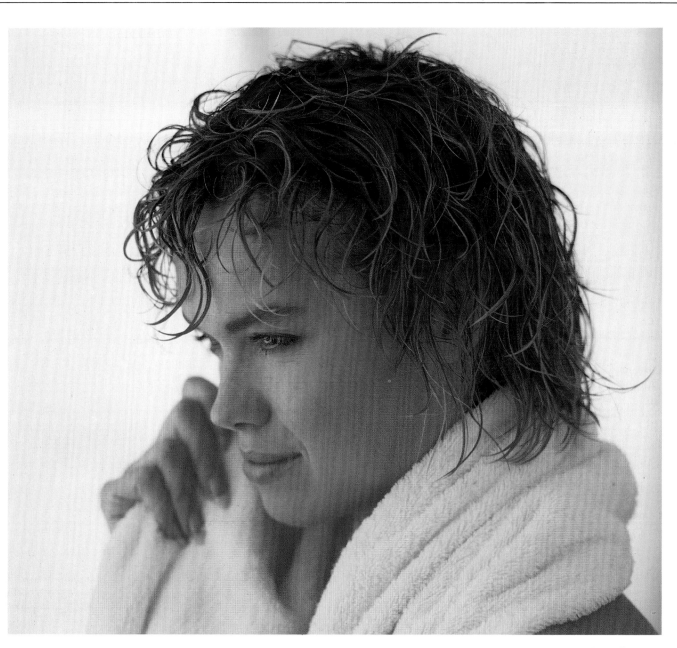

Hair is at its most fragile when wet; that's why it's so important to know how to shampoo, condition, rinse and comb out properly. Always remember to handle wet hair with extra care! (Make-up by Liz Michael, photograph by Chris Craymer).

Believe it or not, the cuticle is also made up of layers, but in this case they are layers of overlapping transparent scales of keratin, which is a hard protective protein also found in the nails on the hands and feet. When the hair is wet these scales open out, and when it is dry they close. Beautiful shiny hair is the result of the cuticles lying smoothly on the surface of the hair shaft where they reflect the light. Dull hair is the product of damaged cuticles which cannot lie flat or catch the light. This kind of hair becomes porous, which

means it absorbs water and other substances at different rates along its lengths.

The second layer of the hair shaft, the cortex, is the main bulk of the hair, and contains the hair pigment granules which give the hair its colour. The medulla is not always present in the hair shaft, but when it is there it is located in the centre and is made up of a soft fibrous keratin.

This may all sound like too much of a biology lesson, but it is important at least to remember that all chemical hair treatments,

whether they be to colour or curl, depend on changes within the hair's molecular structure for their effect. If these treatments are abused, cells in the cortex of the hair may break down, and that is where damage begins. Bear in mind also that, apart from its biological structure, hair is a reflection of our whole well-being, and its condition and growth are influenced by the same factors which affect the rest of our bodies. As we appear to radiate health and energy in the summer, so does hair, and it is a fact that it

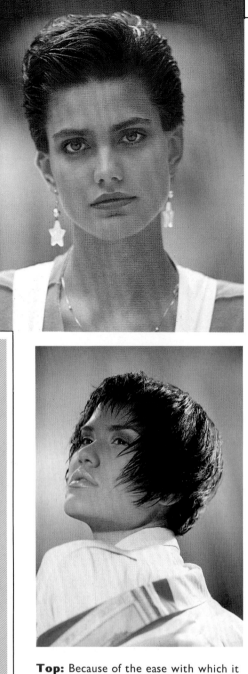

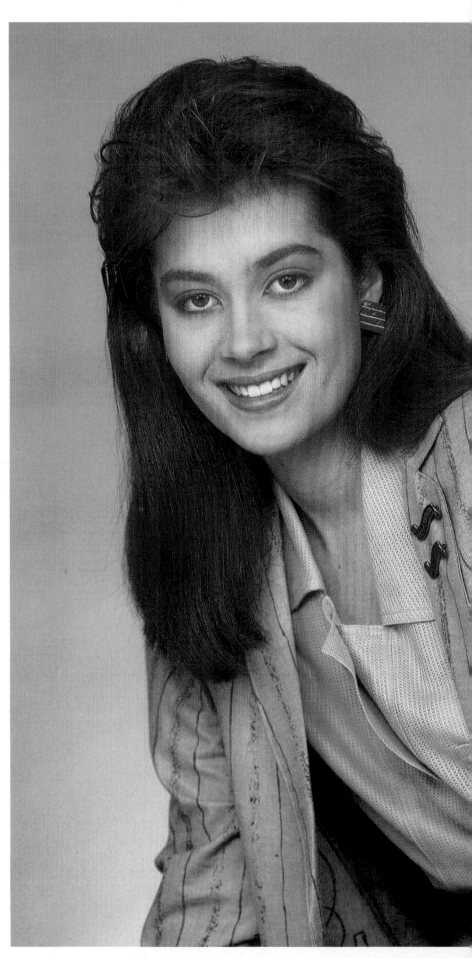

Top: Because of the ease with which it can be handled, short hair has the best chance of being in tip-top condition, as this style from Glemby International shows. **Above:** A super-glossy, face-framing style from Schwarzkopf shows that short hair needn't be blunt to make a statement. **Centre:** Probably one of the most versatile heads of hair —a good length, in superb condition, which can be styled in any number of ways, but which needs careful and regular attention in order to keep its glossy good looks! (Picture courtesy of *Hair & Beauty* magazine). **Opposite top:** Another variation on the timeless bob, which is especially suitable for fine hair (picture courtesy of Schwarzkopf). **Opposite bottom:** No matter what your hair length, a good haircut is always the key to good-looking locks, as this style from stylist John Dacosta illustrates.

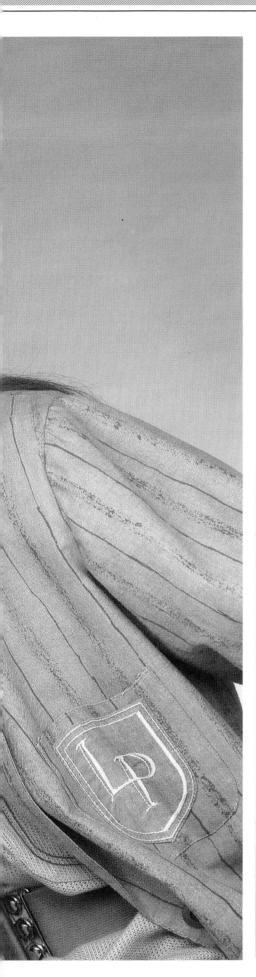

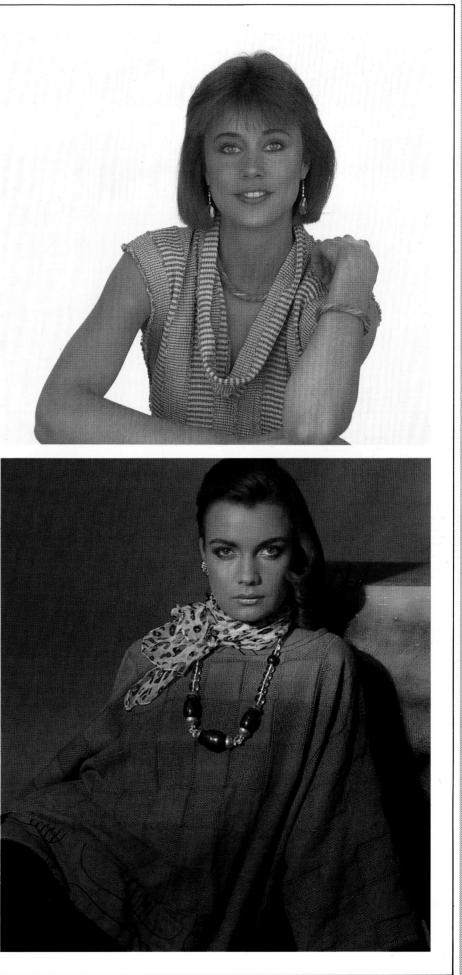

grows faster in summer than in winter. Nutrition affects general body health. Whether we like it or not, we are what we eat, and what we feed our hair is bound to influence its growth. For all this, hair only becomes hair as we know it once its cells have been hardened by the oxygen in the atmosphere and their process is complete. It then becomes dead and we take an interest in it!

Hair growth

Each hair actually lives for between one and six years, grows approximately half an inch a month and completes three phases in its life. It is one of hairdressing's myths that hair grows faster when it has been cut short. It may appear to, simply because growth is more noticeable. That is not to say that a good

cut cannot sometimes make hair appear thicker, and in some cases longer, than it did before.

The first growing phase of a hair's life is the anagen phase, during which normal growth takes place and the papilla is fully active, producing hair cells. The sebaceous gland is also active during this time. Next, the new growth stops, the papilla begins to shrink and the sebaceous gland becomes less active. This is the catagen phase. The final stage in the cycle is the telogen phase, when both the papilla and sebaceous gland become inactive and dormant. They remain this way for a few weeks and then the new hair begins to grow, attaching itself to the old hair which usually remains in the follicle. The cycle takes 80–90 days, the new hair enters the anagen phase and the cycle is repeated. During the telogen phase hundreds of hairs are easily removed by vigorous brushing. All of us lose hair every day; about 100 is quite common and nothing to worry about. It is simply all part of the growth, resting and shedding cycle. Under normal circumstances, 85–95 % of the coarse scalp hairs are in the anagen phase, 1% in the catagen phase, and 4–14% in the telogen phase. With the possible exception of bone marrow, the rate at which hair cells reproduce is greater than that of any other organ in the body. Since the process is so fast, it is easy to see why it is quick to respond to adverse factors such as illness and bad diet.

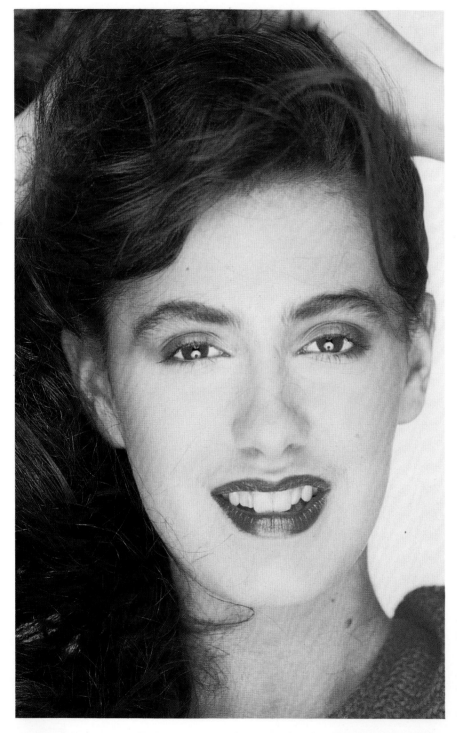

Left: Some hair types naturally do grow much longer, and faster, than others, and it is a fact that hair grows longer in warm sunny climates than in more temperate ones. That's why women in Mediterranean countries always seem to have such long hair (picture courtesy of L'Oréal).
Opposite: An example of just how cleverly hair can be cut and styled to look thicker. This beautiful, bouncy bob is from the Taylor Ferguson Salon in Glasgow.

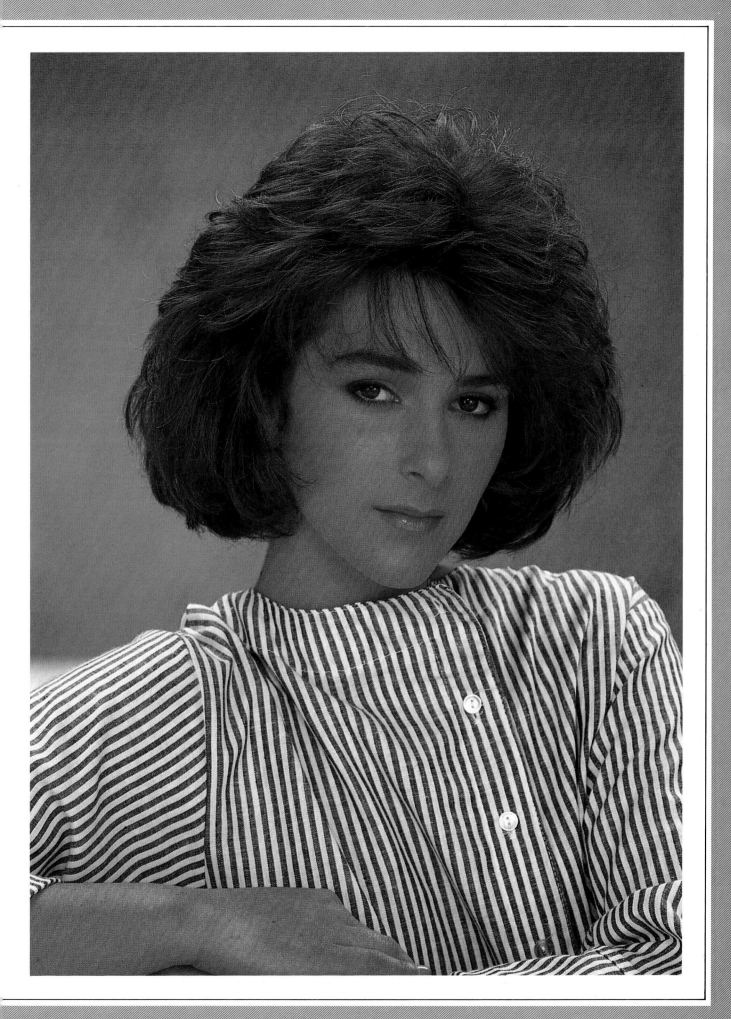

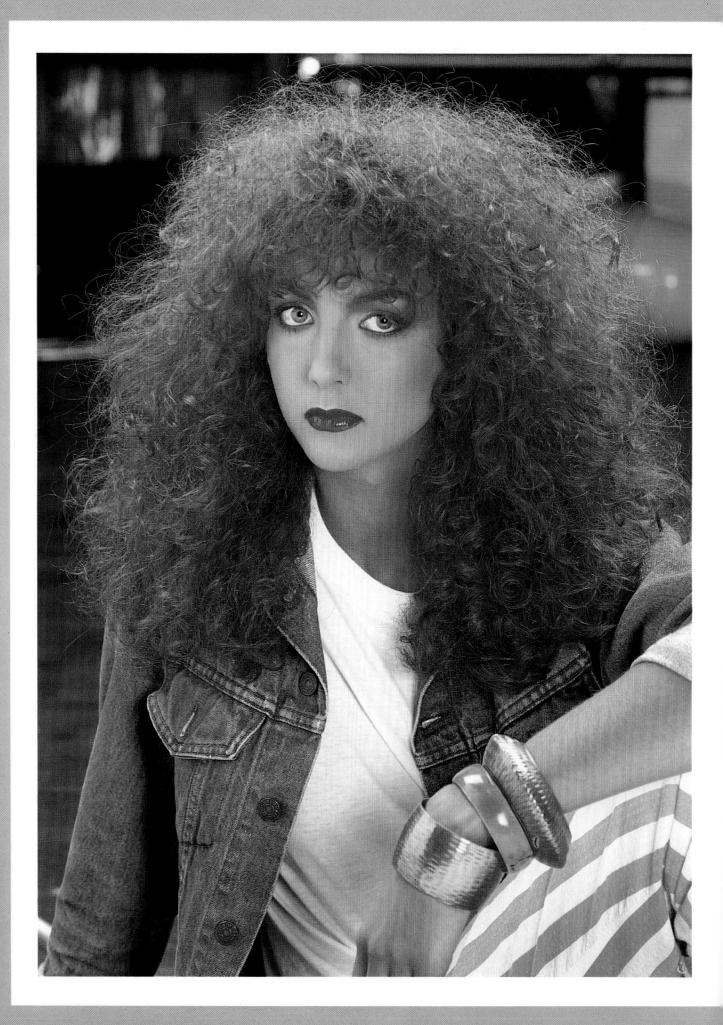

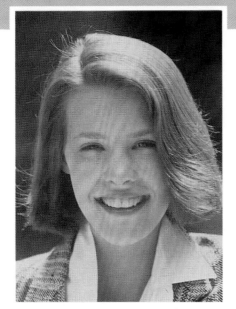

Getting to know your hair

Hair texture and type are as important when selecting a style as the features on your face. If you try to tease your hair into a style it cannot accept, you will only end up by torturing it and yourself.

Hair texture is related to its diameter. Fine hair has a smaller (thinner) diameter than medium hair. Redheads have the fewest strands of all hair types (around 80,000), yet the hair is thick in texture and so appears abundant. Likewise blondes, who have the most strands of hair, often appear to have limp thin hair because it is the finest.

With thick hair the major styling problem is bulk. Layered cuts are generally best because they help to eliminate heaviness and help to tame the hair, making it less wild and unruly. Thin hair is delicate, easily damaged and, sadly, the most common type in Britain. Blunt, simple, short cuts are the best here and a perm can do a lot to enhance a thin head of

Opposite: Naturally curly hair has a tendency to be dry because grease travels faster down straight hair than wavy hair. This beautiful style from Crimpers of London has been handled with loving care. **Above:** A sleek bob on fine hair from Glemby International.

hair – but only if applied under professional conditions, as perm lotions do vary. As for 'normal hair', if it really existed as such it would not be that elusive quality we are all longing to find!

When it comes to hair type, there are anomalies in the scalp which occur in two areas of the dermis, its second layer. These are the sebaceous gland and the blood supply. If the sebaceous gland is functioning normally it will secrete just enough sebum for the needs of the skin. If overactive, it will produce excess sebum, leaving an oily film on the scalp and hair. If underactive, it will not produce enough to meet the requirements of the scalp and hair, thus creating dry hair. The blood supply has the vital job of feeding the hair, skin and sebaceous glands with essential nutrients to nourish, strengthen and give control. If there is an incorrect balance, such as a lack of sulphur in the blood supply, this will cause the sebaceous gland to be overactive.

Generally speaking, if the scalp is greasy the hair will be greasy, and the same can be said of a dry scalp. But if only life were that simple where hair types are concerned! External factors, such as

exposure to the sun and sea without adequate protection, misuse of electrical styling appliances or too much application of heat, can all strip the hair of its natural oils and cause it to dry out. In this case the result could be a greasy scalp with dry hair. But let's deal with each hair type, and a few other common problems, individually.

Greasy hair

We know that greasy hair is due to a lack of sulphur in the blood supply which produces overactive sebaceous glands. The glands become swollen and can increase to three times their normal size, producing excess sebum which causes the hair to become greasy too quickly. Hair is weakened by the continued presence of sebum which prevents it from keratinizing (forming those all-important layers of protein) properly. Oily hair is difficult to manage, lank, lifeless and dull and, without doubt, that is how the rest of you will feel if you don't get to grips with the greases!

It is one of numerous old wives' tales about hair that frequent

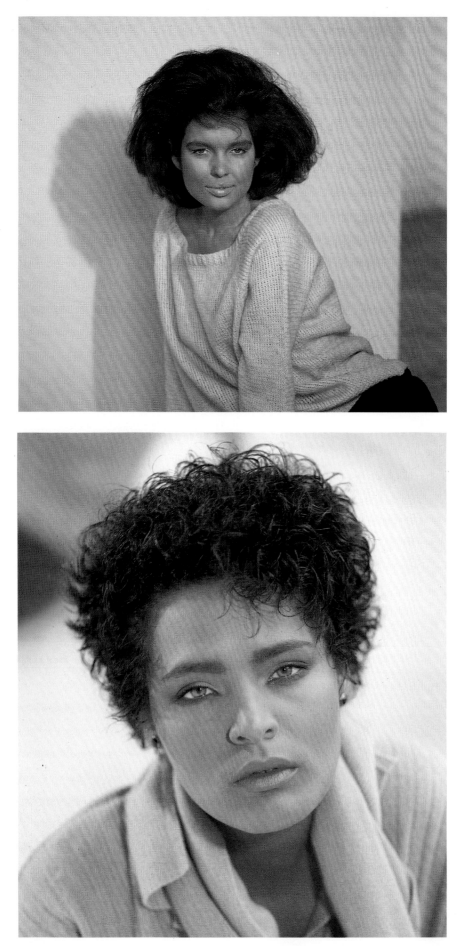

washing will stimulate grease. Greasy hair requires frequent shampooing to keep it clean, but it is important to ensure that you are using the correct shampoo and that you are not stimulating the sebaceous glands by shampooing too energetically. The wrong shampoo used too vigorously will only mean that you are stripping the hair of sebum and, to compensate for its loss, it will produce more. That is where the vicious circle begins. Remember that greasy hair can be controlled but never cured, and watch your diet. Animal fats, oils and starch should be avoided as much as possible. Foods which are good for your hair are good for the rest of your body. You cannot expect to have a healthy head of hair if you are feeding it rubbish. Opt for fresh fruit, vegetables and lean meat – it will do the rest of your body a power of good, too!

Do not use a strongly medicated shampoo but choose one specially formulated for greasy hair which will act as an astringent and help control the grease. When shampooing, always use lukewarm water. Never rub or massage and do not over-lather – the sign of a good shampoo is not in the amount of bubbles it makes. Try using different shampoos, as your hair could build up an immunity to one product.

Keep all styling equipment scrupulously clean – you wouldn't wash your skin with a dirty face cloth. Also, avoid brushing your hair *too much*. In the days before conditioners, and before pollution had become a household word, it may have seemed a good idea to brush the hair with 100 strokes to add lustre and remove surface dirt, but nowadays you will only be lubricating your hair unnecessarily and, in any case, 100

Above left: Layers not only add density to thin hair but make a thick head of hair easier to manage (picture from Schwarzkopf). **Left:** This style from L'Oréal shows just how flattering a perm can be on fine hair.

strokes with the wrong brush could scratch the hair and pull it out.

For an instant lift from the greasy doldrums, try a permanent wave. It will have a drying effect on the hair, as grease travels down straight hair faster than it does down wavy or curly hair. It will also give your hair lift and body, and take away that flat lifeless appearance.

If you want to avoid chemical treatments at all costs, there are a few wise old herbal remedies for greasy hair. The green–grey aromatic herb of southernwood has a reputation for giving fresh life to greasy lank hair if used as a final rinse. A few drops of the essential oil of patchouli, which is a good antiseptic, added to your shampoo are also beneficial for the control of greasy hair. Bay-rum, a popular hair tonic, is an excellent spirit-based lotion for the control of greasy hair. Lemon has never diminished in popularity and it is still associated with products specially formulated for greasy hair – although many of these are just lemon scented. It was not too many years ago that rinses would be made of boiled lemon juice and rind to get that 'squeaky clean' feeling.

Dry hair

Dry hair is brittle in texture and dull in appearance. Its lack of moisture causes cuticle damage and the hair becomes tangled and unmanageable. If your hair and scalp are dry, it is because that all-important sebaceous gland is underactive and is not allowing enough sebum to lubricate either the scalp or the hair. But you may find that you have dry hair and a greasy scalp, in which case the hair has been influenced by external, rather than biological factors.

Heat is one of hair's greatest enemies, and its potential danger cannot be stressed highly enough. Excess heat, whether from misuse

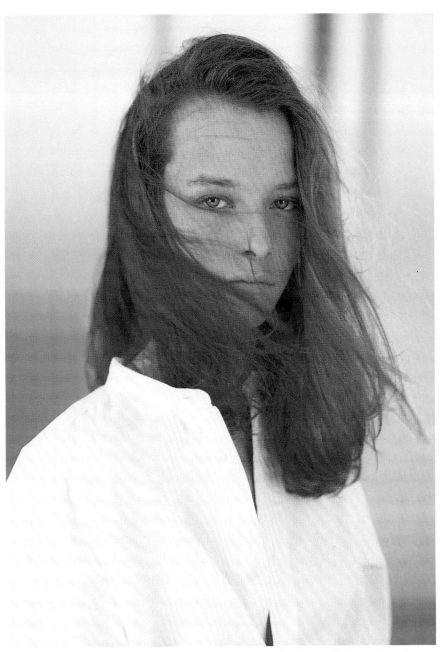

If, like this style from Crimpers, you've got the kind of hair which can be left to dry naturally, you are greatly cutting down on the risk of damage. Heated appliances are among hair's worst enemies.

of hairdryers and electrical styling aids or from too much sun, can damage and dry out hair. Harsh shampoos can wash all the natural oil out of hair. Overuse or misuse of chemical processes such as bleaching, tinting or perming can all make hair dry. If weak, fragile hair has not been treated with the kindness it needs, it too can become broken, damaged and dry through bad handling – misuse of brushes, combs and hair ornaments are great culprits here. You

should make sure your hair is protected from sunlight to prevent further dehydration. You should keep the use of hairdryers and electrical appliances to an absolute minimum. This may mean a change of hairstyle, so seriously consider whether you want an elaborate style of dull lifeless hair or a simple one with hair that appears to exude good health. Another thing to remember is that brushing and combing should be kept to a minimum.

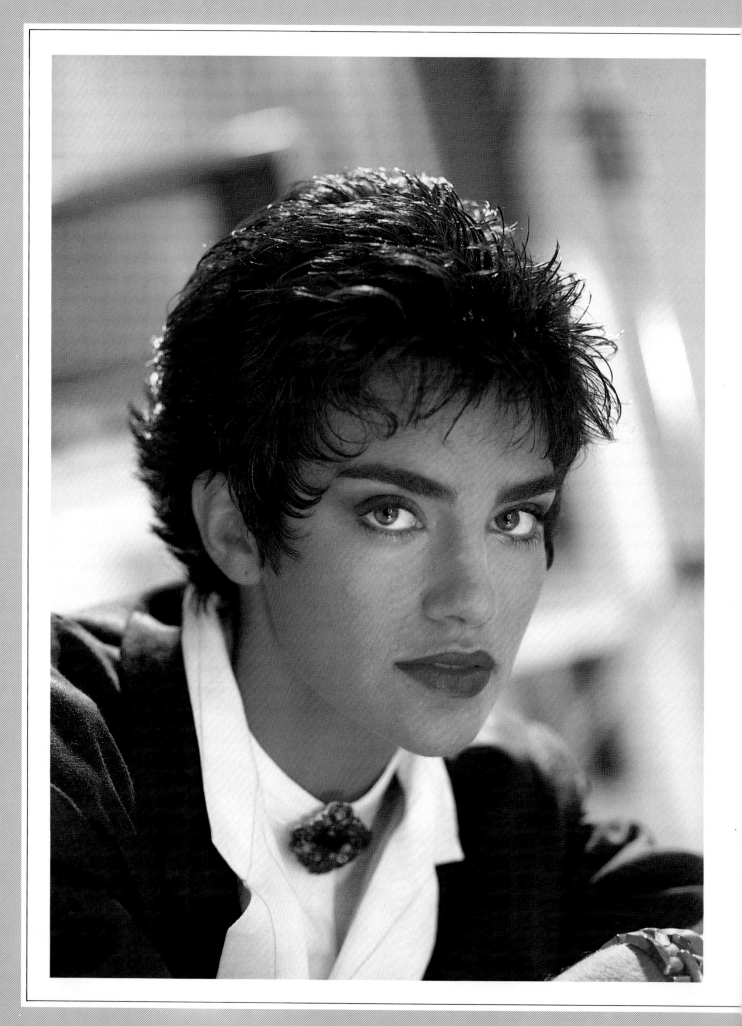

Treatments and conditioning

Dry hair needs to be clean, just as much as its oily counterpart but, before selecting your product, make sure you have established whether your scalp is dry or greasy. If the scalp is dry, the nutrients and lubricants which are not being produced internally need to be replaced externally. Massage is a good idea to encourage the blood to activate the sebaceous glands. A conditioning treatment, at least once a week, is very beneficial for this hair type. Choose an oil-based one and maybe even try working a little warmed olive oil through to the ends of your hair, wrapping your head in a warm towel or cling-film and leaving it on, preferably overnight, before shampooing thoroughly.

If you have a greasy scalp then keep a lookout for a combination product which can treat the hair and the scalp at the same time. Your hair should be regularly conditioned while your scalp is cleansed gently to avoid stimulating the sebaceous gland and causing more grease. Almond provides a light lubricating oil and is useful for nourishing the scalp. A thorough massage with almond oil the night before a shampoo will do much to improve lifeless dull hair. After the massage, and be sure to work well into the roots, the head should be wrapped in a warm towel so that the oil can soak in.

Lavender has a reputation for 'detangling' unmanageable hair, especially if the oil is applied to freshly washed hair before it is combed out. The fragrance is an added bonus with this particular hair treatment! When rubbed into the scalp with the fingertips, the lavender oil acts as an antiseptic lubricant. Rosemary is used

Opposite: Although you can coat your hair with conditioners on the outside, for really healthy hair you need to feed it a healthy diet (picture courtesy of L'Oréal).

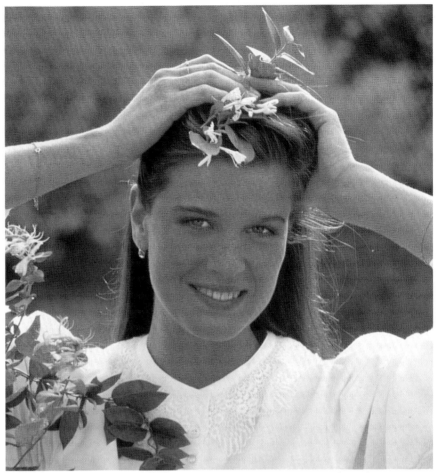

Above: 'Natural' ingredients are used in many shampoo and conditioning products these days, and there are many ways you can treat your hair by using garden produce (photograph courtesy of Yves Rocher).

by herbalists as an ingredient of hair-promoting shampoos, oils and lotions because of its reputation for increasing the activity of the sebaceous glands. In the East, sesame oil is scented with exotic flower perfumes and used as a lotion for coarse, dry hair. Eating sunflower seeds is said to improve the texture and look of lifeless hair and in fact American Indians, with their glossy, dark locks, are known to have used it lavishly.

For moisturizing a dry scalp, try beating together an egg, a tablespoon of vinegar and two tablespoons of vegetable oil just before you are ready to use it. Then massage the mixture well into your scalp and comb through the hair. Leave for 15 minutes (or more), shampoo and rinse well. To make the hair shiny, try whisking together an egg, two tablespoons

of castor oil and one teaspoon of glycerine. Massage the mixture into your scalp and wrap your head in a hot towel. Relax while the towel cools down and then wash your hair thoroughly.

Dandruff

Dandruff is the bane of many people's lives because it cannot be easily disguised. There are 17 known types of dandruff, of which two, dry dandruff and greasy dandruff, are the most common. If it is any consolation, many of us who think we may have this complaint have not really got it at all. What most of us consider to be dandruff is only a flaking scalp, which is false dandruff. This can be caused by numerous things such as too harsh a shampoo used too often, too little brushing, insufficient rinsing, chemical treatments and nervous tension. In the USA people living in cities get more of this kind of dandruff than those who live in small towns and on farms. The reason is thought to be the difference in their lifestyles and the fact that those living in the city endure more emotional stress and hypertension. The treatment for this particular dandruff is simple – use of the correct products – and your hairdresser should be able to recommend the best ones for you.

Few people actually suffer from real dandruff, which is a skin infection caused by the skin's natural antiseptics and defensive mechanisms being overcome by the infectious organisms. Dry dandruff is found on all types of scalp, whereas greasy dandruff is found only on greasy scalps. Dry dandruff is a type of fungus which affects the horny layer, causing it to build up and flake excessively. The flakes fall through to the hair, and the rate of decay of the other layers of the epidermis is also accelerated because of the unnatural disturbance of the growth. Greasy dandruff occurs when the greasiness of the scalp causes the dead skin cells to gather together and become trapped near the roots of the hair. Again, you need a course of medicated treatments to be prescribed, which will usually last five to six weeks to allow the products to penetrate to the level of the germinative layer.

Head lice

People panic at the thought of head lice and automatically associate them with dirt. Yet there is nothing a louse loves more than a clean head of hair in which to nestle down and lay its eggs. As government cutbacks make regular school inspections less routine, head lice are becoming an increasing problem in society today. Head lice are parasites which live off blood. A female will lay her eggs into the hair shaft, and at the same time secrete a cement-like substance which adheres to the eggs very near the scalp. This means that once the egg is hatched, the louse will not have too far to travel to get into the scalp and reach the blood.

Head lice are transmittable by contact and the condition can be treated successfully within days with a lotion or shampoo prescribed by a doctor. Because head lice are contagious it is important that if one member of a family is seen to have them the entire family is treated. Luckily, the very irritation head lice cause means that the problem can be spotted and stopped before it goes too far, but if left it can make a person prone to infection and lethargy – the term 'nitwit' comes from the dozy effect head lice had on their victims in days gone by.

Split ends

In simple terms, split ends occur when hair is 'wearing out' and the individual cell layers of the hair shaft separate. Split ends are a more common problem with long hair than with short, because the longer hair grows the older it becomes. Split ends can also be caused by the age-old enemies, heat and chemicals, and simply by harsh brushing. The only way really to rid yourself of split ends is to cut them off and, to avoid getting them again, don't abuse your hair. If you use an electric hairdryer, set it on medium heat (it should never be too hot anyway, whatever your hair type and condition). Restrict the use of electric curlers to two or three times a week and avoid those with pointed teeth, as they tangle the hair. Use smooth-surfaced or foam rollers, and natural bristle or nylon brushes with smooth edges instead of rough-edged bristles. Comb your hair free of tangles by gently starting at the ends, not near the scalp.

There is a notion that singeing is a cure for split ends, but this is yet another old wives' tale based on the erroneous belief that the entire hair is constantly nourished by a life-giving fluid which flows through a hollow canal in the hair shaft. Cutting, it was thought, would open the end of this canal and release the fluid which would then be lost, causing the hair to die. It was supposed that singeing would weld the hair into a closed point which would act as a stopper to prevent the escape of this vital fluid. We now know that no hollow canal or nourishing fluid exists, and singeing is far more likely to do you harm than good.

Hair loss

Let us begin with the good news – women rarely become bald! It is easy to appreciate why it can be distressing when hair loss does occur, but it is not always a cause for panic. About 15% of the hairs scattered throughout our scalps are going through their resting stage and gradually shedding, and these are the hairs we find on pillows, in the wash basin or left behind on brushes and combs. Only when the rate of loss exceeds the rate of new growth do thinness and balding become apparent. This does happen when people grow older and that is why some permanent thinning of hair is inevitable with age.

There are two kinds of hair loss: permanent and temporary. If it's any consolation to those of you who think you may have a problem, 90% of hair loss is temporary and the situation is self-correcting.

Temporary hair loss is rapid and can be caused by many things. If loss is suffered all over the head it is called alopecia; if in bald patches the size of a ten pence piece, it is known as alopecia areata. Traction alopecia is caused by hair being pulled tight over a long period of time. Constant use of rollers and tight plaiting and frequent styling into pigtails and ponytails can put the hair under severe tension and cause bald spots on the scalp, more commonly along the front where the tension would be greatest. Such loss occurs only after long-term use of these styling methods and not through their occasional use – that's why it's important to maintain hair properly from an early age. It may be quick and neat to drag a little girl's hair back into a ponytail for school, but it could become a styling habit which will only cause damage, and embarrassment, in later years. Most hair lost through traction alopecia will probably regrow, however, because the roots will not have been destroyed.

Postnatal fallout sounds rather a drastic term for hair loss, but it is a common and self-correcting problem. During pregnancy the hor-

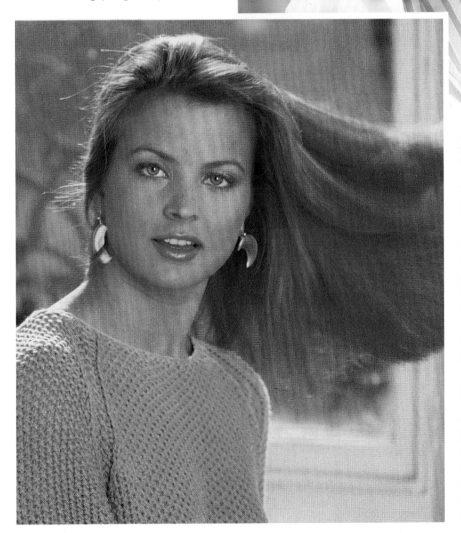

Above: The only way to get around the problem of split ends is to have them cut off (picture courtesy of L'Oréal). **Left:** Even long hair needs regular trimming to keep it in good condition (picture courtesy of Schwarzkopf).

mone progesterone increases and, as nature ensures that she is creating a favourable soil for a healthy body, hair appears to become thicker. This is because the hormones are preventing the hair's normal growth, rest and fallout cycle from taking place. When the baby is born progesterone levels normalize and hair loss occurs. But it is simply the hair which has lain dormant for nine months instead of falling out. Dieting after pregnancy can exacerbate hair loss, and breast-feeding, which ensures that the progesterone levels stay high, delays it. Until the condition

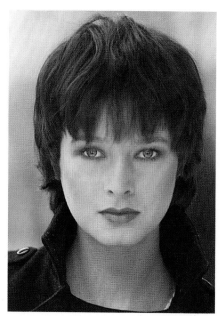

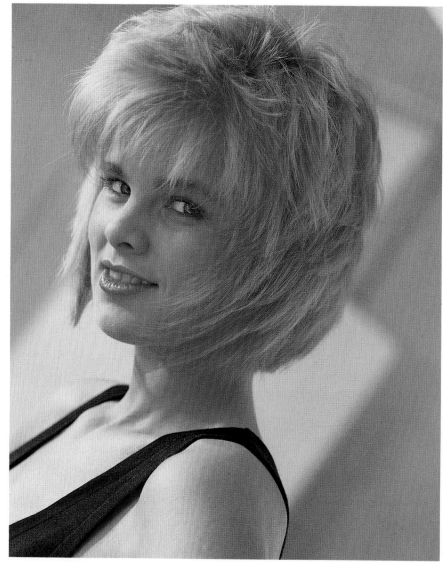

Two styles which require the minimum amount of brushing to keep them looking good. Excess brushing with the wrong tool can not only tear the hair, but can increase the problem of an oily hair type. **Above:** A gamin style from Glemby International. **Right:** Michael Strum of Crimpers designed this one.

corrects itself, manipulate your hair as little as possible. Do not groom it with too harsh a brush but use a soft, natural bristle brush. Shampoo gently with a mild shampoo and pat your hair dry instead of rubbing it. Avoid hairstyles which pull your hair excessively. This advice may not sound too practical to a busy young mum, which is why it pays to invest in a good cut and style before the birth.

The birth control pill can cause mild hair loss for reasons similar to that in pregnancy – hormone imbalance. It is usually only temporary and regrowth generally takes place within several months of a course being discontinued.

There are many other factors which can cause temporary hair loss – illness, certain medications or treatments, dieting, anaemia, thyroid imbalance and stress are among them. Generally speaking, any situation adversely influencing the body's metabolism will contribute to hair loss by increasing the number of hairs in the resting phase of the growth cycle. Hair is

like a barometer of health for the rest of the body and, because it is not vital to its functioning, if something is wrong, very often it will be among the first things the body gets rid of. This is epitomized by the effect that crash diets can have on hair. The body needs carbohydrates for energy so it takes nutrients from other, less important sources – your hair.

Whatever the reason for hair loss, take heart from the fact that it should, eventually, grow back; but expect to wait at least three months before you see any signs of improvement, and check out the cause with your doctor or trichologist so that you can help to prevent it from happening again. There are some deep-seated psychological problems related to

baldness. Trichotillomania is a hair-loss condition among children and some adults. It is a self-inflicted problem caused by the pulling out of large amounts of hair. It can start simply as a nervous habit – a child constantly playing with her hair – or it could be a cry for attention. Whatever the reason, stop it at as early a stage as possible. A child is far more likely to develop this habit at night or while asleep when parents will not be looking. So it's worth an occasional nocturnal visit to the bedroom to keep the problem in check.

As with hair colour and texture, permanent hair loss is something which is determined in the womb, and there is nothing we can do about it. There are two kinds of

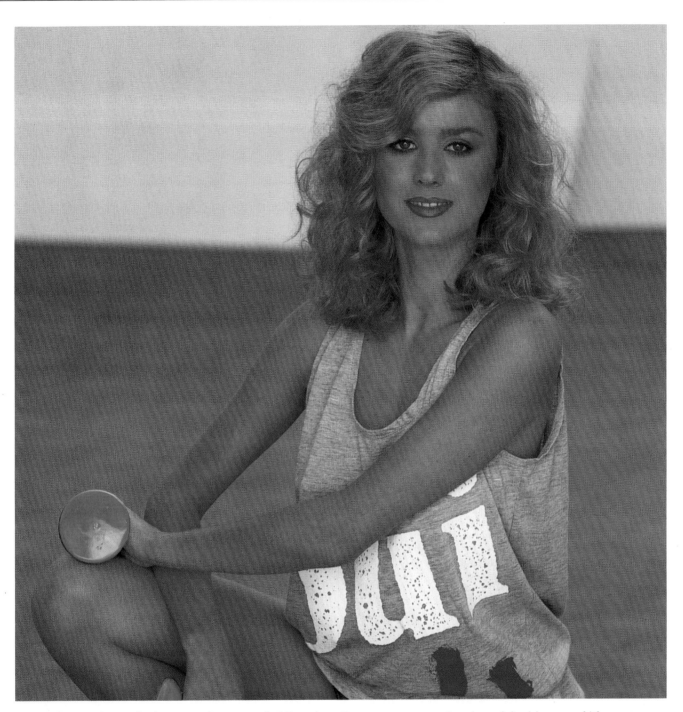

As with most things, the 'you are what you eat' philosophy reflects on your crowning glory. A healthy way of life, as stress-free as possible, and a balanced diet are the best ways of ensuring a head of hair in superb condition (courtesy of L'Oréal).

permanent hair loss though, and the less common one, scarring alopecia, is where the hair follicles have been destroyed through injury or disease. With male pattern baldness (MPB), if there is a history of it in the family, hair loss can even occur in young teenagers. It can sometimes be experienced by women, although not to such an extent – women usually retain sufficient hair to provide adequate cosmetic coverage. The hair growth cycle is important in MPB because the effect of androgen, a common term for the male sex hormone, seems to shorten the growing phase. A man with MPB notices his hair becoming thinner and shorter. Later the hair on top of his head fails to grow to any appreciable length, until finally only a short growth is seen. These short, virtually unseen, hairs are growing from the very roots which originally produced the long, thick hairs of former days.

Male pattern baldness is a sad fact of life. Although research is being done, so far little has been found to improve the situation, and if it is the one thing the man in your life cannot accept he ought to think seriously about wigs and hairpieces.

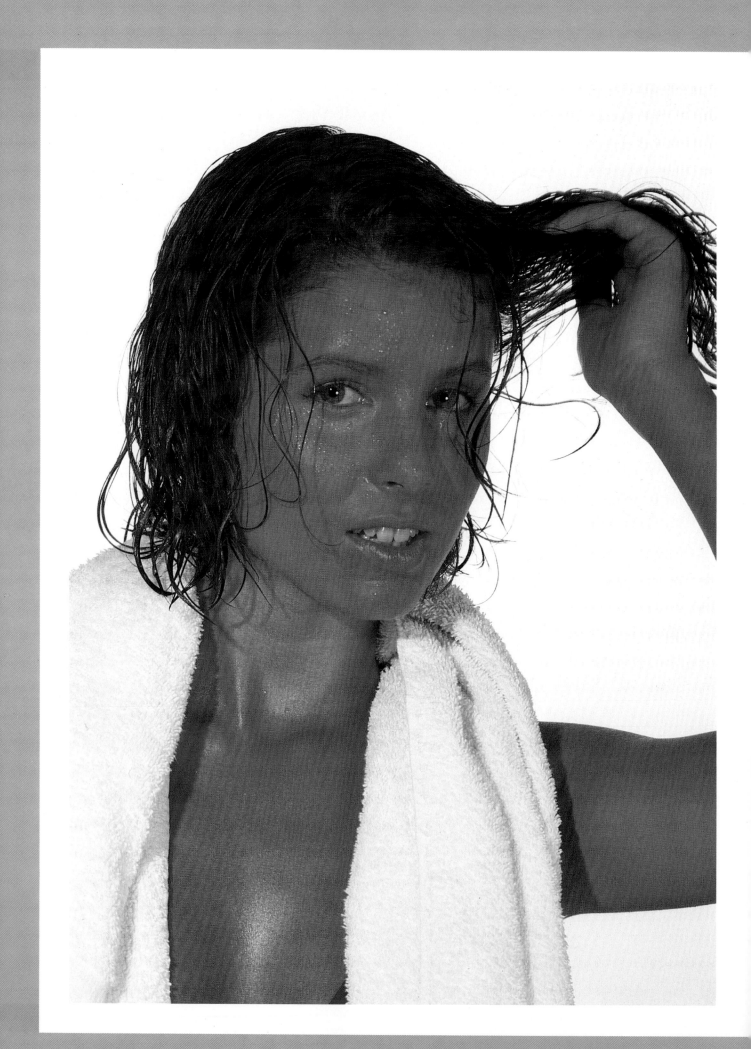

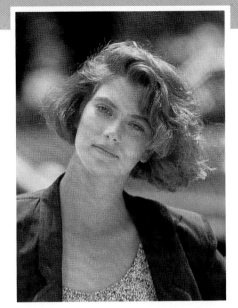

Back to basics

By the time we reach the age of puberty, shampooing is often an everyday task which doesn't get a second thought. We buy products from supermarkets and chemists, usually without any advice on choice, and often make our selection on a bottle's appearance and the fragrance of the contents. Yet shampoo selection should be given as much consideration as any other aspect of our personal hygiene. Continual use of the wrong shampoo can cause no end of damage to hair. But the right product can do a great deal to enhance a style and make the hair exude good health.

Which shampoo?

Shampoo is basically water, detergent and usually some fatty material. The main ingredient is detergent which loosens dirt and grease and cleanses the hair. The most important thing anyone

Opposite: Knowing how to select your shampoo, and how to apply it properly, are crucial aspects of hair care (picture courtesy of Molton Brown, London). **Above:** The right product can really enhance a style (picture courtesy of Glemby International).

should know about a shampoo is how much detergent it contains, but the only way of finding this out is through trial and error, which need not be as expensive a process as it sounds. The best way is to ask your hairdresser. If he has styled your hair for some time he will know its texture and type and be able to advise you on product choice. Any hairdressing salon worth its scissors will stock hair care products for you to buy and use at home, and very often these products are highly professional and are worth the investment of a few pence more. If you have not yet settled on a regular salon and cannot bring yourself to walk into one off the street, then purchase small sachets of shampoo and trial-size bottles until you think you have found the right one for you.

It may also be a good idea to write to a manufacturer or two giving details of your hair type and lifestyle. Most of the major houses will be only too pleased to suggest which of their products they think you should try! Do watch, though, for clever marketing jargon. Some products may claim to have remarkable 'magical' qualities, which they probably do, but in such small quantities that they can

hardly affect the condition of your hair at all.

Buying a shampoo for one particular hair type is a bit like reading a horoscope; it applies generally to so many thousands of people that only a few can possibly find it a perfect match for them. Hair, like personalities and star signs, changes so much from one individual to another. Remember, too, that the detergent in a shampoo loosens dirt and oil and washes them away, so any other ingredients in the shampoo are not going to stay on your hair but end up down the drain with the dirt and oil!

Many shampoos today are pH balanced. This means that they have the same pH as hair, and so do not change its natural pH. The term pH means potential hydrogen; it indicates the concentration of hydrogen in a solution, and is a rating of the acidity or alkalinity of a substance, on a scale of 0–14. The middle of the scale is 7, and this is the point at which acidity and alkalinity balance each other out so that the solution is neutral. Distilled water has a neutral pH. The numbers 0–6.9 indicate acidity, and 7.1–14 represent alkalinity.

Skin and hair are acidic. They have a pH of 4.5–5.5. Shampoos are either alkaline or acid-balanced, so if you have many chemical treatments using alkaline products you should be using an acid-balanced shampoo.

Dry shampoos are used less and less these days, as frequent washing becomes more acceptable, but in cases of illness or lack of time they can be a godsend for occasional use. While dry shampoos don't clean hair as thoroughly as wet shampoos do, they at least remove some surface oils, dirt and odours.

There are a few points to bear in mind when selecting a shampoo. If you are washing your hair more than twice a week, the chances are you don't need more than one lather, so your shampoo should be able to cleanse your scalp and hair thoroughly with only one application. Remember that the amount of lather means very little. Some shampoos which produce little lather cleanse the hair extremely well; hair should be left looking soft, shiny and manageable. The shampoo must rinse off easily, it must not be irritating, and it must be simple to apply. Lastly, you have got to enjoy using it! If you have to live with the bottle in your bathroom for a few weeks, make sure that you like the colour, perfume and texture of a product.

This is not meant to make you wary of buying hair care products altogether – far from it. It's merely to advise you of the factors to consider when selecting them – what's good for your best friend is not necessarily ideal for you. There are shampoos you can make yourself at home, which will not be as convenient or as scientifically based as those you can buy, but they could be fun to try.

Do-it-yourself shampoos

First of all, you have to know how to make an infusion. Just pour one pint of boiling water over one ounce of herbs (whichever you select), then put a lid on the container you are using and keep it warm; leave it for three hours. Strain the liquid into a tight-lidded jar or bottle and keep cool until it is required.

For starters, try making an infusion of camomile, rosemary or sage and add a cupful to your regular shampoo. Wash your hair in warm water, then for the final rinse use cold distilled or purified water (some people find sparkling mineral water especially invigorating!). The properties of camomile are good for enhancing blond hair, whereas sage and rosemary are good for dark hair.

To exploit fully the versatility of eggs, try cracking a few of them into your hair care routine. For a basic egg-yolk shampoo, beat two egg yolks into a cup of warm water. Massage into your scalp and hair for five minutes and leave for ten minutes, then rinse thoroughly.

If you have light-coloured hair, make a strong infusion of camomile flowers. If your hair tends to be oily, add an egg white beaten to a froth; if it tends to be dry, add an egg yolk. For dark hair, replace camomile with sage or rosemary.

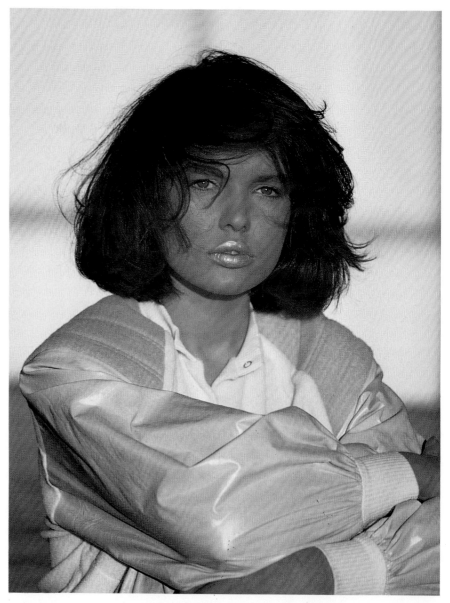

Above: Rosemary and sage are especially good for enhancing dark hair (picture courtesy of Schwarzkopf). **Opposite:** Camomile brings out the best in blond hair (picture courtesy of *Hair & Beauty* magazine).

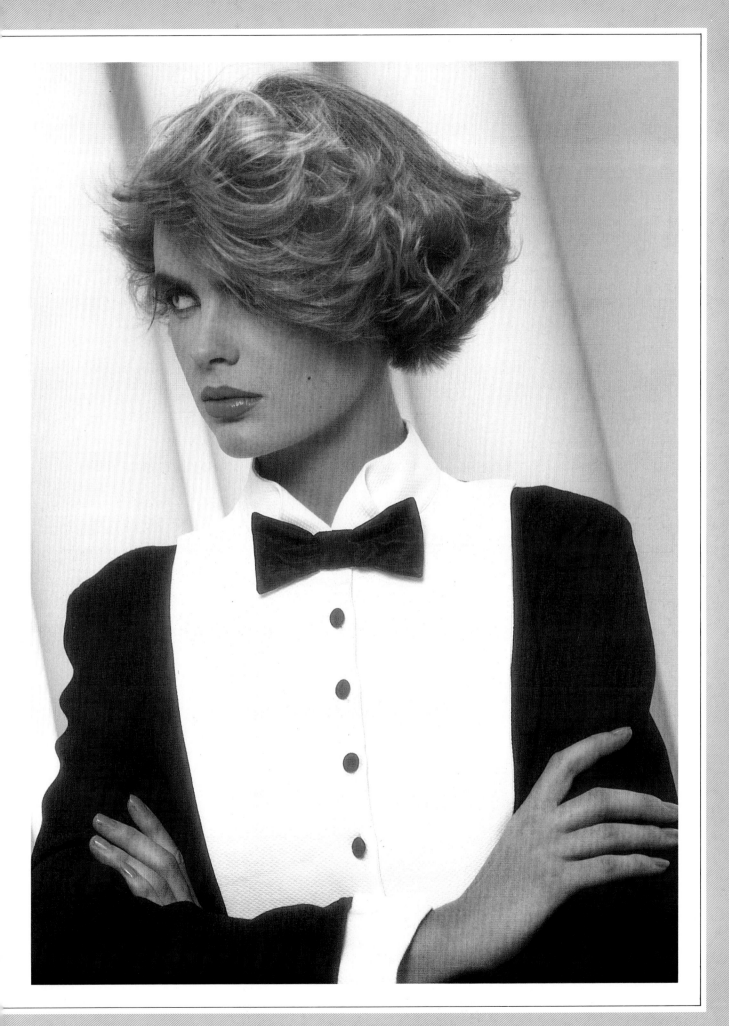

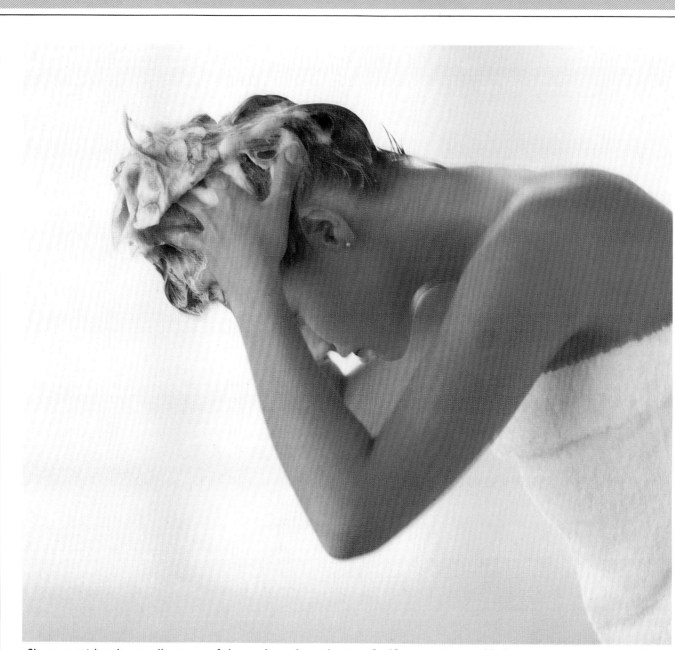

Shampoo with only a small amount of the product, about the size of a 10 pence piece, and lather up gently — remember that lots of lather doesn't necessarily make for a better shampoo. Always be sure to rinse well (picture courtesy of Vitapointe).

How to shampoo

Now have a good think about your shampoo routine. If what you do is to apply liberally a good dollop of shampoo straight on to the head, then you need to go back to basics. First of all, wherever possible, you should wash your hair with a hand-held shower or spray. You cannot possibly get your hair clean in the bath, when the water you are using is dirty. If it is just not practical to use anything other than the bath, rinse your hair afterwards with fresh water.

Brush the hair free of surface dirt before you begin. Apply a small amount of shampoo, roughly the area of a teaspoon or ten pence piece, on to the palm of your hand and gently massage it into a lather with your fingertips. Work on the scalp rather than rubbing the hair, and make sure you remember all those areas which can so easily be neglected — behind the ears, the back of the neck and the hairline. It cannot be stressed too highly how vital a part rinsing plays in your washing routine. When you think you have rinsed your hair

thoroughly, do it all over again, once more paying attention to those parts of your head which are not so easy to get at. If shampoo is not rinsed out properly it can cause irritation and dandruff, and your hair will not really be clean at all. At all stages of washing, try to keep the water temperature warm rather than hot. Apart from being uncomfortable, too high a temperature will stimulate greasy hair.

Conditioners

Conditioning is nowadays as automatic a part of any hair care regime as shampooing, but all too often conditioning is used as a blanket word when it means entirely different things. Think about what you are doing next time you reach for the bottle. As the hair we wash is dead, there is not a great deal we can do to revive its condition, except to re-think our diet and the treatment of our hair, and wait for a few months to see the results on the new hair which grows. But we can cheat with our hair's appearance and use conditioners to put on the gloss. There are, however, various types of conditioner and the intensive, protein conditioning treatments we should all use regularly will be dealt with in a later chapter. For now we will look at creme rinses, or instant conditioners, which are the kind we use after each shampoo and are designed to help make the hair easier to comb, to reduce static and generally to leave it looking good and more manageable.

After-wash conditioners help to flatten the keratin layers of the hair shaft so that they overlap each other. This gives the hair a smooth, sleek appearance. You should be using about the same amount of conditioner as shampoo (roughly the area of a ten pence piece). Apply it after the final shampoo and rinse – usually after the hair has been slightly towel-dried, but products do vary and it always pays to read the instructions. It should be poured *not* directly on to your hair but on to the palm of your hand, and you should gently spread it over the other palm before distributing the conditioner over the hair. Remember that conditioner is for the hair, not for the scalp. Massage it in from underneath and work all over the head. If your hair is particularly oily or if you wash it every day, it may not be necessary to apply conditioner after every

wash and, when you do, only to the very ends. Leave it on for a couple of minutes before rinsing off gently with lukewarm water. For some conditioners it is recommended that you comb them through before rinsing, but do remember that wet hair is very fragile, so always handle it with care.

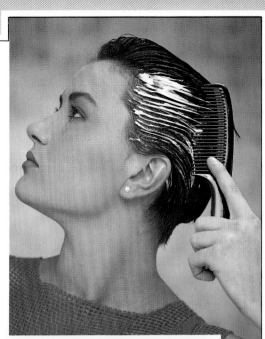

Right: Wide-toothed combs are the kindest to use on wet hair. One was used to apply a conditioning mousse to the hair when wet in this picture.
Below: A light, feathery, finished result (pictures courtesy of Schwarzkopf).

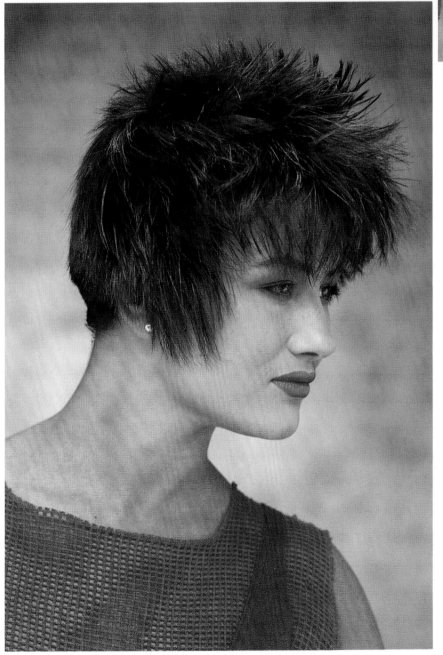

Drying

It is when you are styling and drying your hair that most damage is likely to occur. Heat is the worst possible enemy your hair can ever have and, if you are tempted to aim a hot dryer too close to the hair, bear in mind that you are probably releasing enough energy to fry an egg. That kind of intense heat will damage your hair irreparably. Moreover, you will never, ever, get your style to look remotely like it did in the salon if you apply too much heat too close to the head – the style will simply collapse. Always lightly towel-dry your hair first to get rid of excess moisture. Hand-drying techniques will be dealt with later, but it helps to do as much with your hands to get the hair past that initial soaking-wet stage before applying any heat. Remember never to brush your hair when wet. Always use a wide-toothed comb which will get it gently and neatly into place without tearing it. When you are actually drying the hair, use a nozzle on the hairdryer to protect it and keep the dryer moving. Don't concentrate on any particular section for too long and always keep the dryer at least six inches away from the head.

If your hair is very flat and limp and you need a little more volume, try going through the initial rough drying period with your head upside down. Armed with your styling brush in one hand and dryer in the other, you can now start to style. You will have to pull the hair slightly as you style in a direction away from where you want the finished wave or curl to be. Concentrate the dryer for a few moments up and down the particular strand or section of hair you are styling, keeping the stream of heat moving all the time, and allow the hair to cool off before removing the brush. Finally, allow the hair to cool before brushing the style through.

Before we deal with the more complex subjects of selecting a salon, and a style, which are right for you, let us go over a few basic home hair care hints.

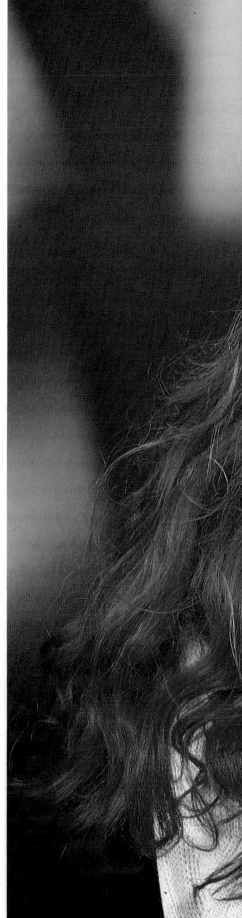

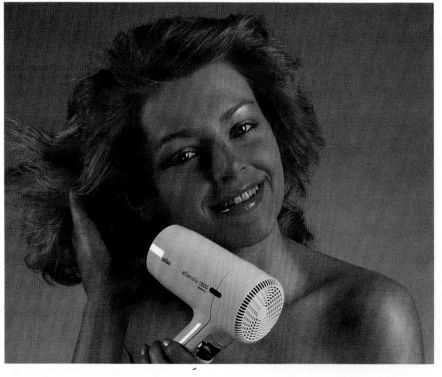

When using a hair dryer, never have the setting too hot and hold the appliance a fair distance away from the hair (picture courtesy of Braun).

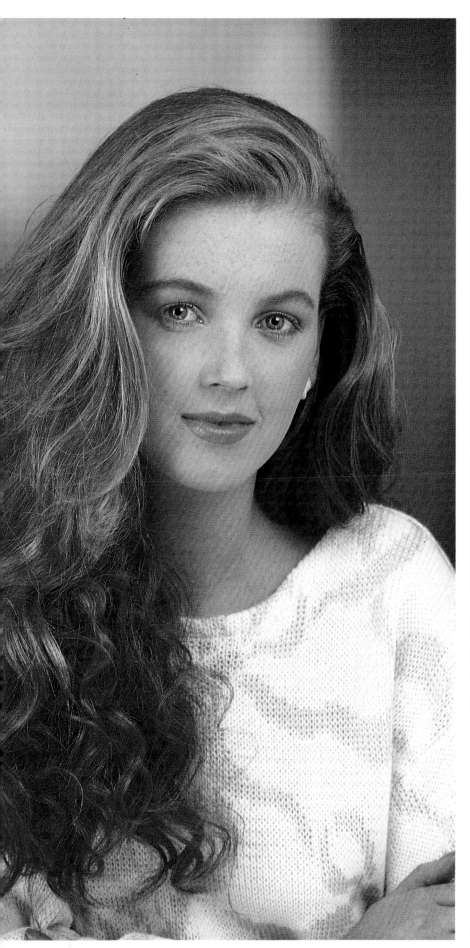

1 A ten-pence sized blob of shampoo, and conditioner, is sufficient.

2 Don't judge a shampoo by its lather; it's not the foaming agent in a product that cleans your hair.

3 Rinse your hair thoroughly after every shampoo, otherwise it will look limp and dull after only a couple of hours.

4 There's nothing wrong with washing your hair every day, even if it is very greasy, but make sure you are using the right products and are not stimulating already over-active sebaceous glands.

5 Hot water will only make greasy hair worse, so always rinse with cool water.

6 Don't treat your hair roughly after shampooing. Gently pat dry with a towel to absorb excess water.

7 Don't start to blow-dry your hair when it's still dripping wet.

8 If you need extra volume, try drying your hair with your head upside down and running your fingers through it from the roots during the initial drying stages.

Fairly confident that you are now at least cleaning and taking care of your hair properly, you can go in search of what some consider to be that elusive person – the perfect hairdresser for you!

Left: Long hair needs special care, especially when washing, drying and grooming. But the result, a healthy head of long hair, always pays dividends. L'Oréal helped groom this naturally curly head of hair.

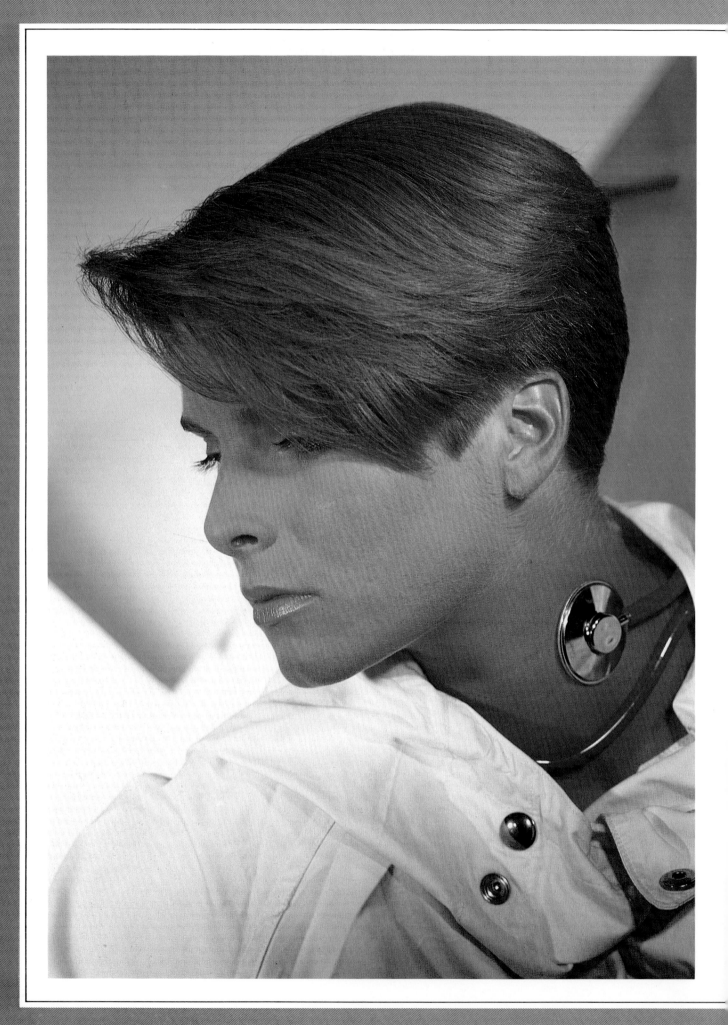

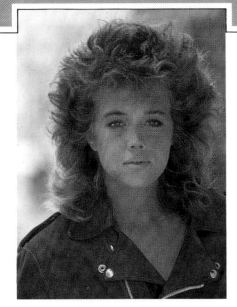

Style counsel

Which salon?

For many of us, good hairdressers are precious treasures and friends for life. They are hailed as being miracle workers and are followed, almost, to the ends of the earth. There are also those of us who believe, perhaps as the result of bad past experiences, that hairdressers are out to chop off our locks and be done with us, that they don't care a snip about us as people and that good, caring hairdressers are a figment of glossy media imagination. Well, they *do* exist and nowhere more profusely in the 1980s than in Britain. British hairdressers are held to be among the best in the world, and not just because of their creative talents, which are plentiful enough.

In the 1980s, hairdressers have had to become astute businessmen in order to survive and, in doing so, have realized that, more than

No matter what your preference, somewhere out there a salon and a hairdresser are waiting for you.
Opposite: A first-class precision cut (picture courtesy of Schwarzkopf).
Above: A shaggy perm makes a mid-length style adaptable (picture courtesy of Glemby International).

ever before, the client must come first; there is no room for prima donnas. They have become caring professionals, and a good hairdresser will nowadays be as happy to snip off half an inch as he will to create a totally new headline-hitting style – as long as he is satisfied that that is what the client wants. For each of us there is a tailor-made hairdresser, if not several, out there somewhere. To find him or her we have to break down the initial barrier, the salon.

It may be that you have to experiment with several salons before finding the right one but, even if this is the case, never select a salon in haste. It pays to do a little groundwork first, and one of the best ways to ensure that you are at least going in the right direction is to ask other people. If you see someone in the street or in a shop with a style you particularly like, ask where their hair was done. The person will be flattered, and if you hit upon the same salon after two or three enquiries you know you are on to a good thing.

The best salons are inevitably the most profitable ones. If a salon is successful it will make money, and it can only do this by pleasing

its clients time and time again. That means building up a regular clientele and giving them what they want. So look for a busy, clean salon which is also geared towards retail sales. This doesn't necessarily mean earrings, make-up and sweatshirts, which can sometimes play such a prominent part in a shop front that you hardly know it's a salon at all! But selling shampoo and conditioning products to be used at home are all part of the completely professional service which good hairdressers now offer. After all, they don't want to create a beautiful look one week and see you wandering around the streets, your hair limp and lifeless, the next!

The fundamental rule is that, whichever salon you choose, you have got to feel comfortable in it. It's no good going into an ultra-chic hairdressers with a first-class reputation if you feel like a fish out of water. If you do you will never communicate properly with your stylist and, as a result, you will never be happy with the service. Communication is the key to finding the right hairdresser, and the salon environment should

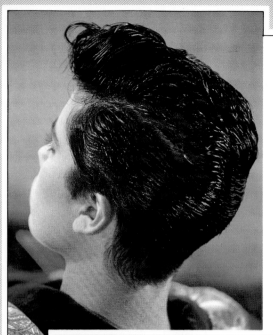

infuse you with enough confidence to enable you to talk openly about yourself.

A good salon will be clean, friendly, efficient and sometimes chaotic, but it should be organized chaos! You should receive a warm welcome from *someone* the moment you walk through the door. If the person at the reception desk does not acknow-

Left and below: Lawrence Falk at Crimpers created this excellent short, sporty cut. Although the back looks boyish, the front can easily look more feminine by using styling aids.

ledge you with at least a nod within a few moments of your entering, even if he or she is on the telephone, then you will start to wonder what you are doing there and your confidence will evaporate. If it is your first visit and this happens, then think twice about whether or not you want to stay. You should be an important person to yourself and to your future stylist, and it isn't right that you should pay to be ignored. A good hairdresser will swot up the appointments book first thing in the morning and have at least a vague idea of who is coming in.

Choosing a stylist

If you select a salon because of someone's name above the door, try to find out first with a phone call the days on which that person is in the salon and go along then. It's not that anything disastrous is likely to happen if the owner isn't present, but staff do tend to be more on their toes and inspired when the boss is around. If you are at all nervous, that knowledge will help your confidence along a bit. Problem number one is solved: you have opted for a particular salon and you now need to make an appointment. But who with? If you have asked around before trying a salon you probably have a name in mind, but if you are totally clueless the obvious person to consult is the receptionist. Tell the receptionist what you want. It may not, for example, be necessary to have the top stylist if the cut you require is a simple one. If you would prefer a male hairdresser to a female one, then *say so*; it isn't the time to be humble. If you really need more convincing to ensure you are in the right hands, just make an appointment for a conditioning treatment or a blow-dry of your current style. When you are actually in the salon you can tell for yourself whose work and personality you like best of all.

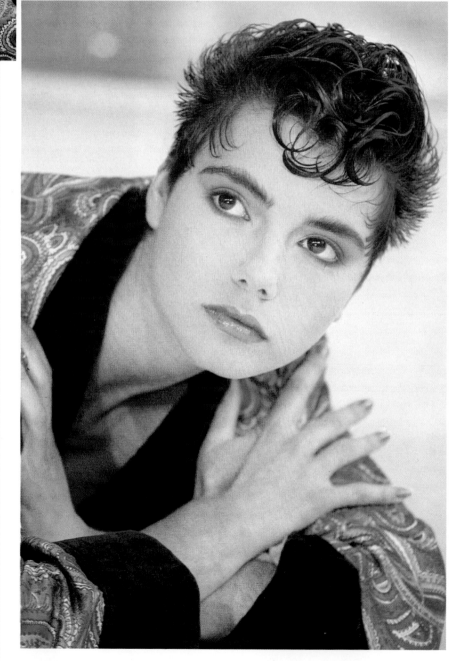

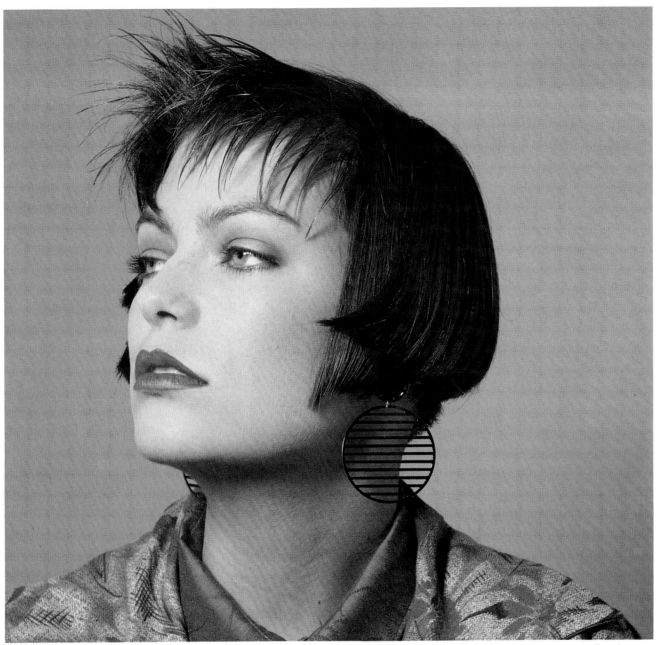

The focal point of this model's style, her fringe, easily updates the whole appearance of a short, classic cut, as well as her entire image. This picture from Schwarzkopf again shows how easy it is to have a short but adaptable hair style.

Communication

You really cannot be too familiar with your hairdresser! Building up a relationship with your stylist is like building a friendship. The more he or she knows about you the longer that relationship will last, and the better and more fulfilling it will be for both of you. Believe it or not, hairdressers really do have clients they hate because they never seem happy. What a blow it would be if you were one of them! So *communicate*. Salons sometimes offer initial consultations before appointments. If yours does, take advantage of it. Relax, be yourself, and tell the stylist what you want. Honesty is the best policy. If you are nervous, shy or tense then let it show. A good hairdresser will not want to hurt you by changing your appearance too radically all at once. He would much rather build up your confidence bit by bit. After all, he knows you are in his salon because you were not happy with your previous one, or did not have one at all, so he is going to do his utmost to please.

Always go to the salon dressed the way you most enjoy looking, as a true reflection of the way you see yourself. If that means donning full make-up and an expensive outfit, then do so. It's all part of telling the truth, being yourself, and communicating. If your stylist has only two minutes to assess your personality before you sit in his chair, your appearance is going to do a great deal to help him.

If you really are tongue-tied and know what you want but just cannot explain it, then take along pictures from magazines. Far from being frowned upon, this is an ideal way of showing a stylist what kind of look you want to achieve. What may be short and spiky in your eyes may not, after all, be so extreme to a hairdresser. He will probably want to push you to your limit in style and fashion awareness – so make sure, by whatever means you can, that he knows what that limit is! Let the stylist know, too, how you feel about yourself. Do you hate your nose but feel your eyes could be emphasized? Do you like your ears showing and would you rather your forehead were covered? Are you shy or outrageous? Do you really prefer short hair or are you essentially a long-hair person? How much time are you prepared to spend on your hair every day? Do you play sports frequently?

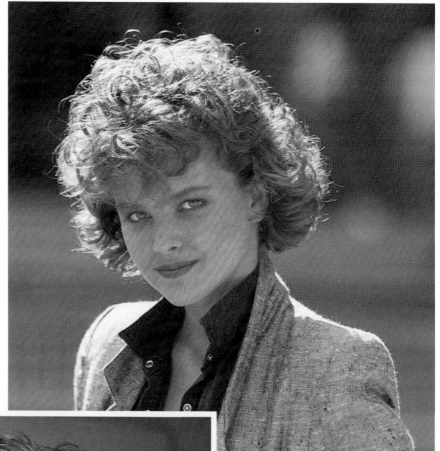

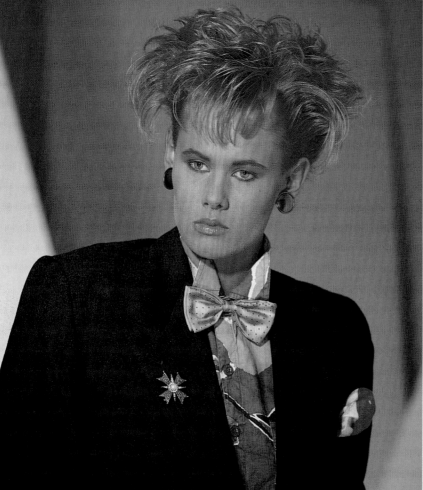

Your hairstyle should be created to match not only your face shape, but your lifestyle and your personality. **Above:** A pleasant, curly style from Glemby International. **Left:** Hair is boldy styled high using gel by Michael Strum at Crimpers.

Face shapes

All of the above factors, which should help result in a style which enhances your personality and total appearance, are vitally important when considering a hairstyle, but stylists still have to bear in mind certain facial features. The style in which you have your hair should emphasize your best features and disguise or minimize your worst. Faces tend to fall into several basic shape categories – diamond, heart, square, oblong, round, pear and oval. If you are lucky enough to have an oval face your hair will be easier to style because almost anything will suit you. But the other face shapes need more consideration.

Diamond

The diamond-shaped face is characterized by a narrow chin and forehead and wide cheekbones. Fullness or width are needed in the forehead, the hairline and the lower cheekbone area of the face. Fullness is not needed in the area of the upper cheekbones, and the hair should be styled close to the head in that area. A fringe is a good idea for disguising a narrow forehead, and fullness around the jawbone helps to create an oval illusion.

Heart

If you have a large, wide forehead and a narrow chin then you have a heart-shaped face. By bringing hair on to the forehead you will reduce the area across it. A pageboy-type style is good for the lower sides of the face because the hair is close to the head at the eyes, where narrowness is needed, but slightly full towards the face around the jaw and below and in front of the ear lobes, where width is needed.

Square

A square-shaped face is the result of a wide hairline and jaw. In this case it helps to create that much sought-after oval illusion by bringing the hair forward and close to the face just below the cheekbones, and setting and combing the hair off the forehead. This also has the effect of adding height to the face. You can break the wide, straight lines of a square face by combing hair on to the sides.

Oblong

Oblong faces are characterized by a very long and narrow bone structure, and people with such faces often have long, thin necks as well. A fringe across the forehead, accompanied by soft waves or curls across the crown and nape, is flattering to this shape of face.

Round

Your face is round if you have a wide hairline and fullness at and below the cheekbones. Your neck may also appear short. Creating height in the top and crown sections of the hair can diminish some of this roundness.

Pear

Pear facial shapes are those with small or narrow foreheads and a large pouch-like jawline. It is a good idea here to style the hair so that it adds width from eye level through to the crown area of the head.

Spectacles

If you wear spectacles, don't fall into the trap of hiding under your hair. With the variety of frames available these days there's no excuse for not finding a pair, or several, that you actually enjoy wearing. Make a fashion feature of them and emphasize your eyes rather than disguise them. Take your hair *away* from your face, and let your features do your talking for you.

Last of all, remember that communication is a two-way thing, so listen to what your stylist is saying. He sees enough clients every week to tell whether or not a certain look is going to work and if he says pointedly, 'Are you absolutely sure?', then think again. You can bet your bottom dollar that he or she is trying to tell you, as politely as possible, that the style for which you have been longing for months is not going to suit you at all.

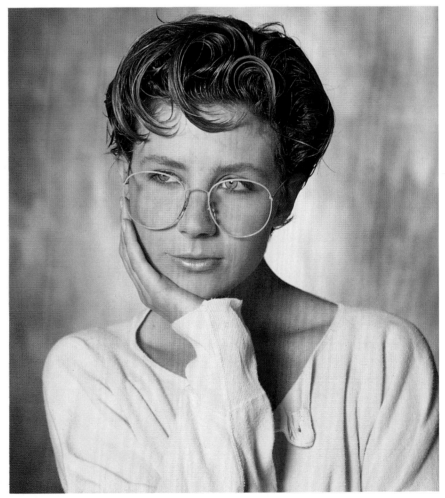

If you have to wear spectacles, choose a hairstyle to complement them (photograph courtesy of Pearle Vision Ltd).

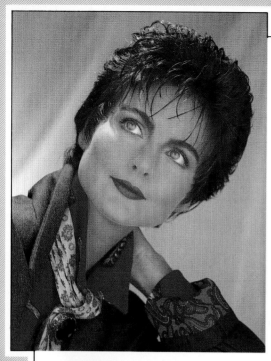

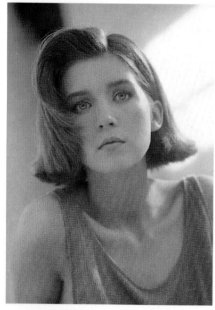

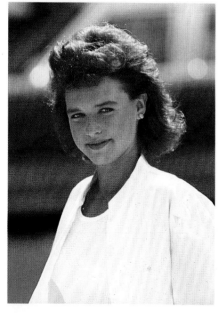

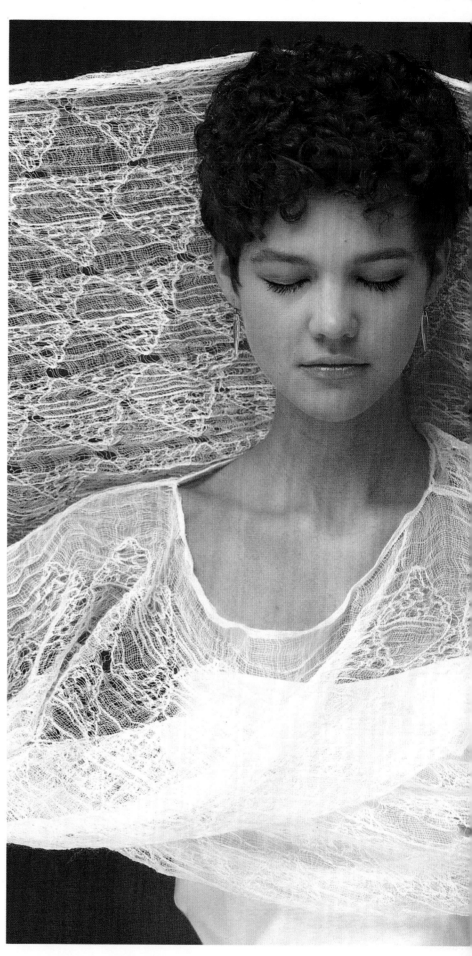

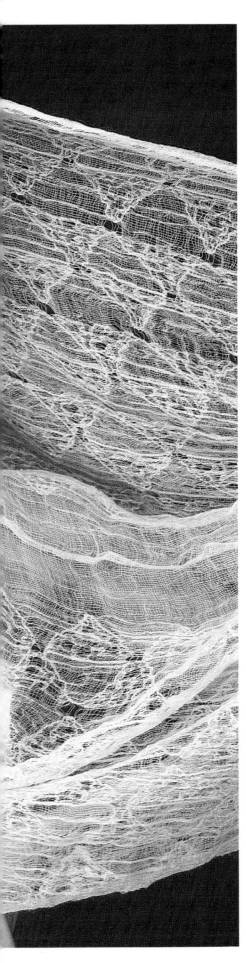

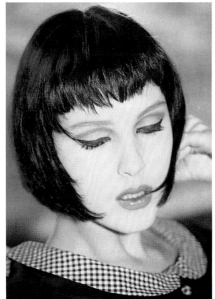

Opposite top: It's a good idea to style hair on a pear-shaped face so that it adds width from the eyes to the crown (hair by the Stevie Buckle Salon, London). **Opposite centre:** Hair brought on to a square face just below the cheekbones helps to create an oval illusion (hair by L'Oréal). **Opposite bottom:** This soft style from Glemby International helps to create fullness on the forehead and lower cheekbone areas of a diamond-shaped face. **Centre:** This picture from Molton Brown shows how a round face can be made to appear less so by creating height on top of the head. **Left:** This picture from Schwarzkopf illustrates how the wide forehead of a heart-shaped face is reduced if hair is brought across it. This adds much-needed width to the jawline. **Below:** A long face is flattered by a fringe and soft waves (picture courtesy of L'Oréal).

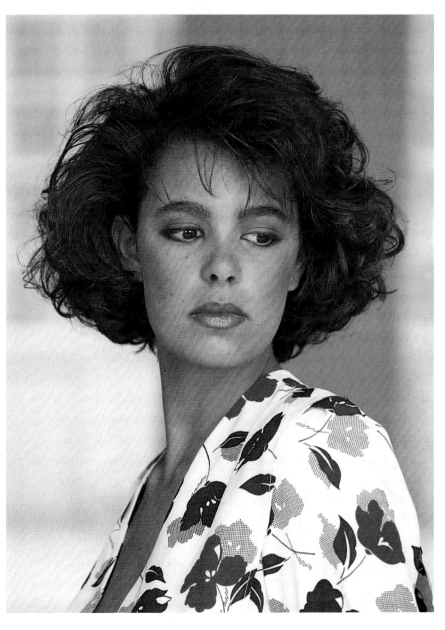

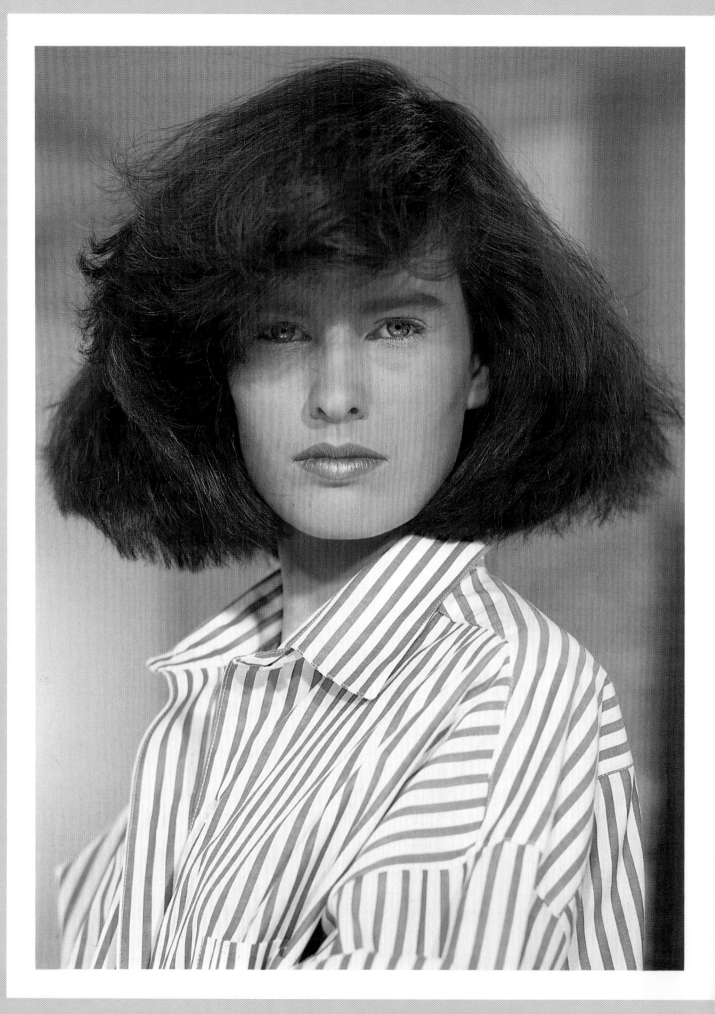

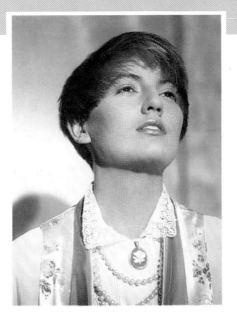

Sensational styling at home

Having got a style you were more than happy with in the salon, it can be agonizing to go home and find that you simply cannot get it to look anything like as good yourself, no matter how hard you try. As the tears of anger and frustration well up, that's when many of us decide to change salons or swear blind we will never go to a hairdresser again.

Styling techniques have never been so varied and they really are not all that difficult to perfect, but before we go on to talk in detail about the masterful art of styling, do remember that your hairdresser is providing a service; exploit it. Don't just watch him style your hair or flick idly through a magazine while he dries it; *ask* him how best you can do it yourself. It's one thing for a hairdresser, who after all has the advantage of both hands free and all-round vision, to make it look superb within five minutes. It's quite another for you to blunder

Opposite: Michael Strum at Crimpers shows how a style can be kind to the hair but still stunning. This one was finger-dried to save using a hairbrush. **Above:** This sleek style was blow-dried, using a hand-held dryer and a brush (by Lawrence Falk at Crimpers).

your way through at home and end up in tears. The most common mistake that anyone ever makes with their own hair is that they try too hard. A good cut on a suitable head of hair really will sit the right way all by itself, and if you are teasing it inexpertly in another direction it is bound to rebel.

Styling terms

First of all, let's cut through the jargon used by hairdressers and in magazines to describe some of the more innovative, and popular, drying terms so that you have at least a vague idea of what your stylist is talking about!

Blow-drying is the most widely used home-styling technique and has been popular now for something like 15 years. It's simply a method of using a hand-held dryer, with a nozzle, and a brush to achieve a certain sleek look.

Scrunch-drying is for more casual looks and is achieved by crushing, in a clenched fist, damp-to-nearly-dry hair.

Finger-drying is when you use your fingers as if they were a brush, creating movement by air distribution through the hair and

pushing it into place. It is similar to finger-waving where, by using a comb and your fingers, you can form the hair into waves.

Rough-drying is another method of achieving a casual, tousled look, which can be done by tipping the head over the knees and drying the hair away from the head as opposed to towards it.

Scrub-drying is a method of scrubbing the hair with a vent-type brush and rotational-drying is when the hair is dried in circular movements with the palm of the hand.

Styling aids

Most drying techniques rely heavily on the use of styling aids for manageability and to help maintain the styles. Nowadays, when it comes to setting your hair in place, anything can and does go. But those aids which have developed and played a more prominent part in hairdressing in recent years are setting lotions, hair sprays, mousses and gels.

Setting lotions very rarely feature as prominently in salon dressing-out units as they once did, but are still widely used. They

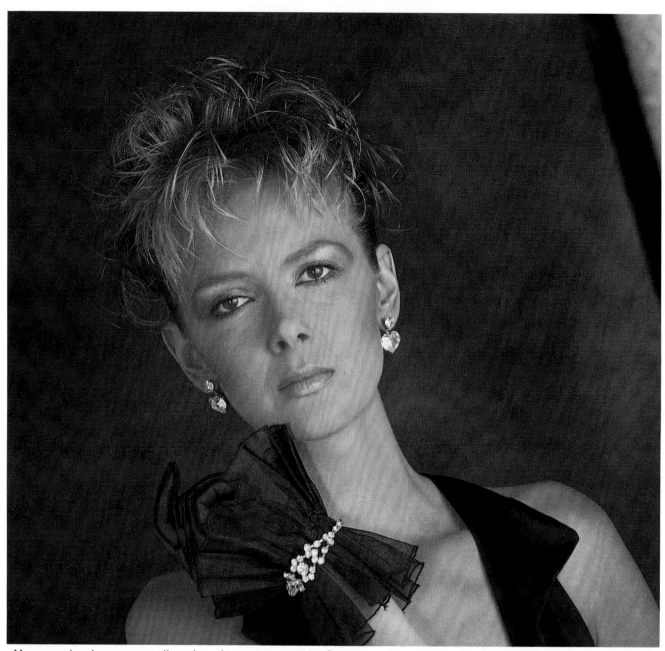

Mousse, gel and spray were all used on this evening style by Christine at Mane Line in London. A deliberately casual evening look which contrasts well with glamorous evening wear, it was finished off by being finger-dried on top.

became fashionable with the advent of permanent waving, and are designed to make the setting of hair easier and to preserve style and tidiness. They are liquid, and therefore runny to apply, so sprinkle the lotion over all the hair ends, lengths and roots after the hair has been shampooed and towel-dried. Work it through the hair as you apply it and comb through before setting.

Hair sprays are very thin, quick-drying varnishes which can be sprayed on to the finished hair-style, or on to a brush or comb and then worked through the hair, leaving a transparent, flexible film of resinous material which helps to preserve the set of the hair and imparts to it a lustrous sheen. After styling dry hair, spray lightly, holding the can 10–12 inches away. If more volume is needed, brush the hair forward, spray the roots and then smooth back into place.

Mousses have really taken the hair fashion industry by storm in the 1980s, and are surely the most popular form of styling aid available. Mousse is a hair-thickening agent which adds gentle body and volume to the hair. It comes in aerosol cans and has a thick, foamy consistency – which makes it easy to apply. Most mousses are suitable for all types of hair and, because some have conditioning agents, can act as a protective barrier against harmful effects of hairdryers and heated appliances. They are especially good for curly hair as they give it body and shine and make it slightly oily (curly hair

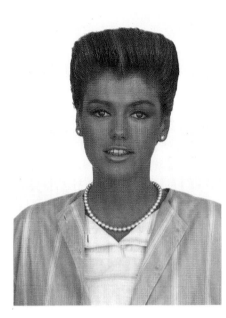

tends to be dry). They also stop hair from going frizzy and separate the curls.

Mousse is designed as an aid to drying, so apply it to damp (but not soaking wet) hair. Shake the can well and squirt a blob of mousse on to the palm of your hand. The amount you need will depend on the length and thickness of your hair, so whereas a quantity the size of an egg will be

Left and below: Schwarzkopf did a double-take of this style to show just how much can be done with hair. **Left:** Short and sweet and not a hair out of place. **Below:** Mousse was used for extra body and bounce when drying the hair.

sufficient for a short style, you will need more if your hair is long or thick. Apply the mousse all over your head with your fingertips, working it out from the roots to the tips. Mousses can also be used on dry hair, perhaps to control frizziness, as an end-of-the-day pick-me-up to a hairstyle, or even to give a tired style temporary bounce until the next shampoo.

Mousses do vary in texture and effect. If the one your hairdresser uses on your hair seems to work perfectly, ask him what it is and try it at home. Generally speaking though, the stronger the hold, the stickier the mousse will be. Mousses are a convenient as well as a fun beauty aid because the cans fit snugly into handbags. Moreover, they don't leak and, because they are easily transportable, can be taken on holiday.

Gels offer no soft options. They are clear, concentrated formulations which hold the hair and give it a sheen. They can be used to sleek down hair for a smooth or 'wet' look or to make it stand up for spiky styles which appear totally to defy gravity. Rub a blob of gel between warmed palms, and apply a little at a time, using fingers to work through dry or damp hair. It is important to use a little, rather than a lot, at a time to make full use of the gel's build-up potential. If your hair is fine, apply gel only at the roots to avoid weighing down your locks and, to help get to grips with frizzy hair, smooth a little gel over the surface of the hair when it is dry. Too strong a gel or mousse can make hair dull and dry. To find out how strong it is, put a small amount on the palm of one hand and press your hands together. If they don't come apart easily, the product is strong — use it on wetter hair to dilute it.

Mousses and gels are a boon to any girl's dressing table. Not only are they quick and easy to use, but with a little imagination they can add variety of style to one cut — even a very short one.

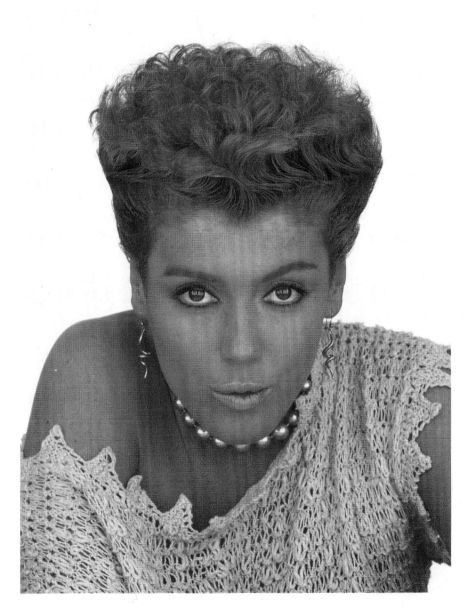

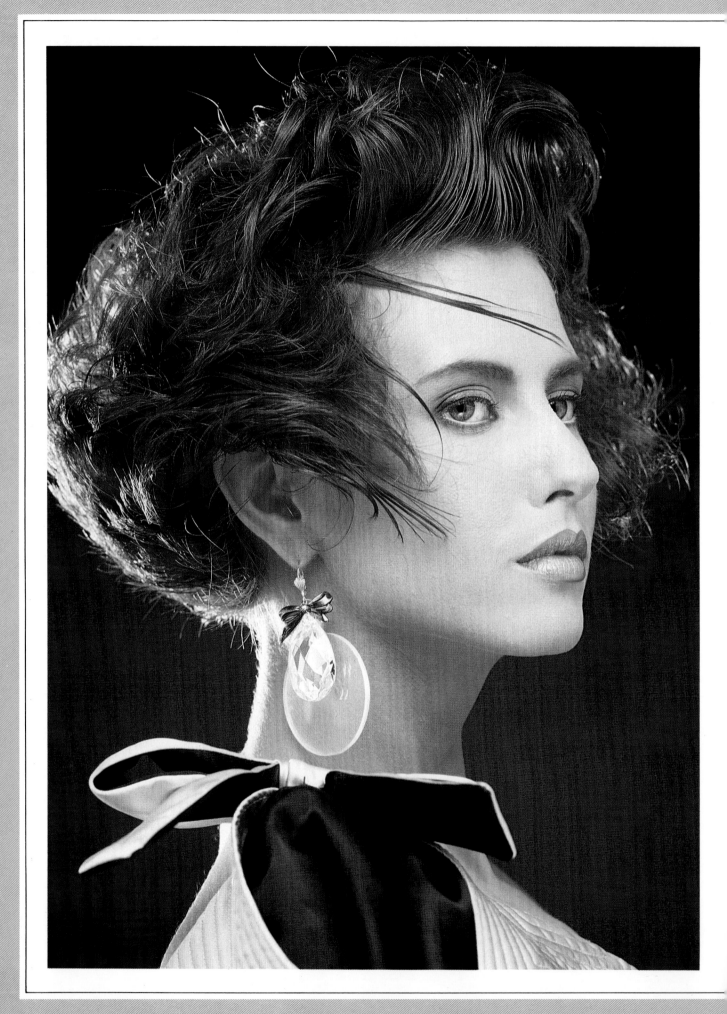

Opposite: Which way the wind blows! An example of just how many directions hair can have, all at the same time, from Crimpers of London. Practice with styling aids can easily create a look like this. **Right:** Permed hair can still need a little coaxing into place, and this style was helped along the way with a little styling glaze (by Kervin Murphy International for Alberto TRESemme). **Far right:** Gel is usually preferred for sleeker, more upright looks. This one, from Schwarzkopf, needed a little spray to keep it in place. **Below:** Even hair which doesn't defy gravity can still benefit from a helping hand with styling aids. Gel was used to complete this look by Michael Strum at Crimpers.

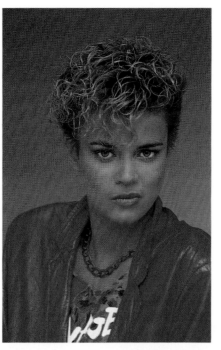

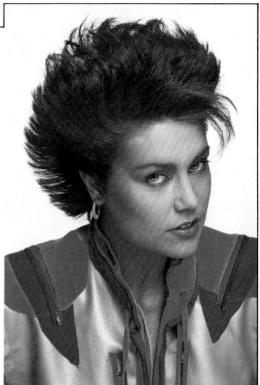

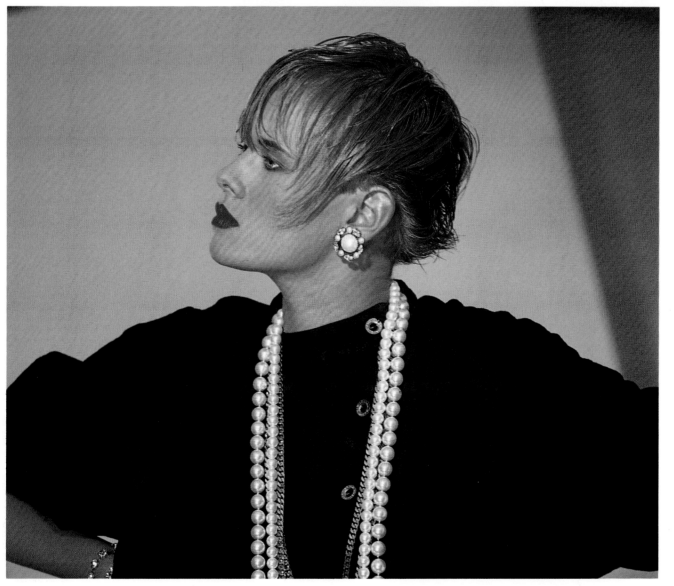

Methods of drying

Despite all these magical styling aids, you still have to be pretty adept at drying your hair to achieve exactly the look you want. If you really cannot stand the thought of getting to grips with a hairdryer and styling brush or a can of mousse, you should opt for a wash-and-leave style which virtually takes care of itself.

If your hair is shoulder length or longer, your main problem will be dealing with bulk and it is important to section the hair in some way so that you don't attempt to dry too much at once. These days you will rarely see a hairdresser painstakingly sectioning each part of your head and clipping it with sectioning clips. Modern drying techniques are much faster and just as effective, and if you see the stylist fiddling with numerous grips you will inevitably feel that you will never be able to get it right yourself; with patience you will, but you will also need to glean as much information as you can from your hairdresser, to get a good haircut, and to practise.

No matter what your particular drying technique may be, never be tempted to start with a soaking wet head of hair; it will take twice as long to dry and end up looking limp and flat. Give it a good towel-dry or rough dry with your hairdryer to remove excess water. Don't make the mistake of drying the front of your hair first. It may seem more convenient but it means that the back will never behave; by the time you get round to it, it will have dried quite stubbornly in its own way. Try doing a straightforward parting down the middle at the back of your head and drying from there, gradually working your way round on both sides until you get to the front. It's the way in which the roots of your hair are dried that gives the style direction, so don't be tempted to concentrate on the fiddly little bits at the end and neglect the area near your scalp – the style will just drop out.

Blow-drying

Blow-drying is the art of using a hand-held dryer and brush to create casual styles with volume. Before you start practising with your styling equipment, it's a good idea to tilt the hair forward while it's still wet and blow-dry it roughly in an upward direction from the roots. This will help remove excess water and add more volume to the style. Then take a small section of hair at a time from the nape and wind it around the brush of your choice (a small, radial brush will achieve a tight curl and a larger brush a straighter look). Wind the hair either under or over the brush, depending on the look you want to achieve. You need to pull the hair slightly as you dry it around the brush, in a direction away from where you want the finished curl to be. Keep the dryer on a cool-to-warm temperature setting. If the heat is too strong for your skin then it is certainly too

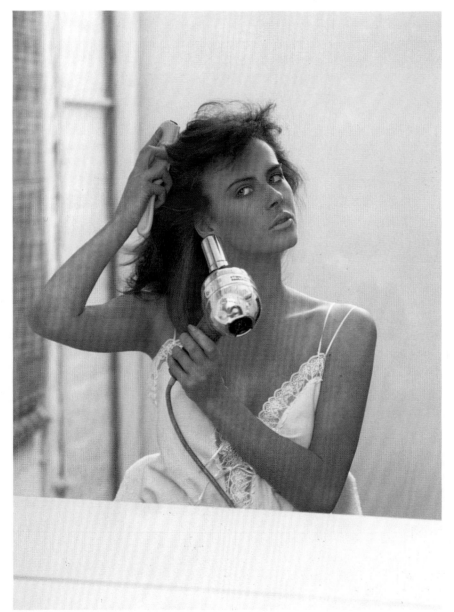

Left: Never be tempted to blow-dry your hair on too high a heat setting or too close to the head; your hair will be damaged and your style quick to drop out (picture courtesy of Vitapointe). **Opposite:** A sleek style which has been blow-dried (picture courtesy of Philips and *Hair Flair* magazine).

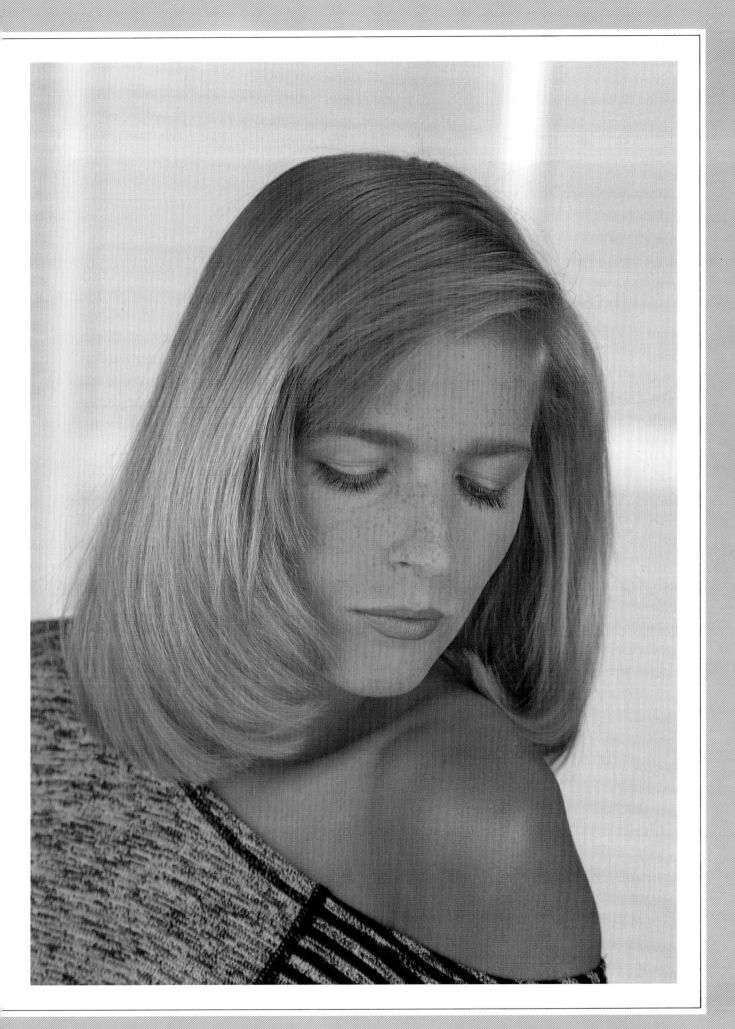

strong for your hair. Keep the dryer moving over the brush and don't concentrate for too long on one area – you can always go back to it once it has had time to cool down. Allow a few seconds for the hair to cool off before removing the brush. Dry the hair this way all over until you are certain it is dry – if you leave the hair slightly damp the style will only fall out. Leave the hair to cool for a short while before you brush or comb through.

Scrunch-drying

Scrunch-drying is one of the most popular styling methods in use. It is simple and quick yet can achieve some quite dramatic looks. This technique depends on the hands and fingertips to create body and curve, and the process can be speeded up with the use of a hand-held dryer.

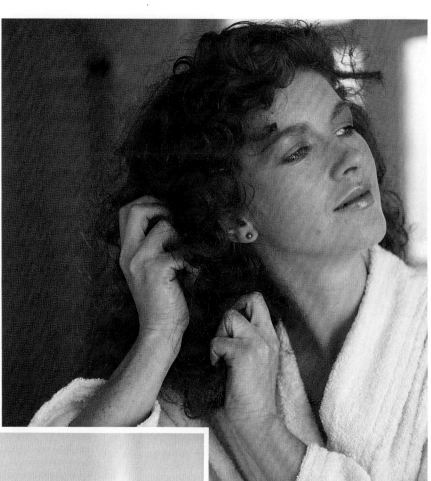

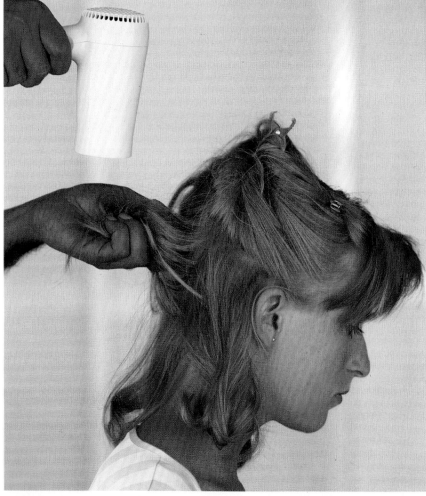

Above: Scrunch drying is a quick and easy way of achieving a dramatic look; it depends on the hands and fingertips to create body and curl (picture courtesy of Vitapointe). **Left:** Scrunch drying using a dryer fitted with a detachable nozzle adds extra body and texture to the back and sides (picture courtesy of Philips and *Hair Flair* magazine).

Begin with towel-dried hair and don't comb it through. Instead, arrange it roughly with your fingers into the shape and direction you are after, gently untangling any knotty problems as you go. If you are going to use a styling aid, now is the time to work it through your hair. Take handfuls of hair and scrunch them in your fist, relaxing and letting go. Use the palms of your hands to push hair up away from the scalp, and use your fingers to separate each curl or wave. Rub each strand of hair between the fingertips to remove moisture and build shape.

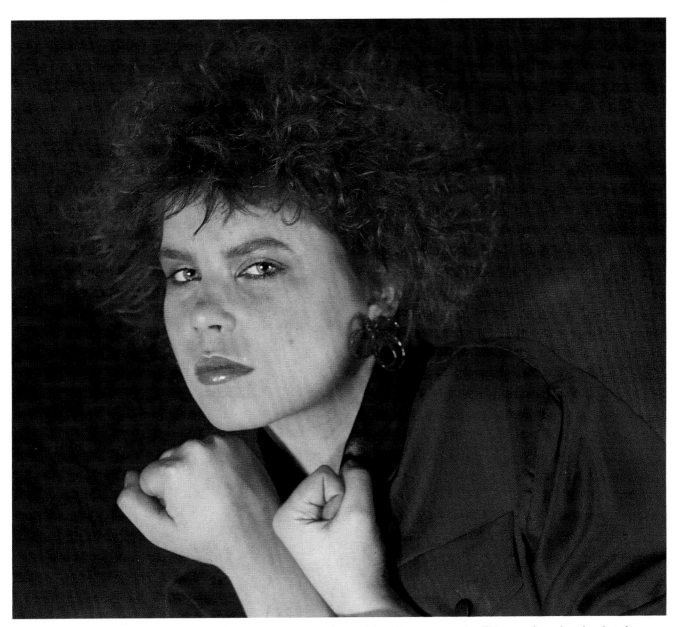

The art of scrunch drying lies in quick, decisive movements; be positive about your style. This one, from London hairdresser John Dacosta, shows just how scrunch drying can be used to create whatever style fashion dictates.

All this is done with quick, decisive movements. Be positive about your style and don't fuss or fiddle.

Setting

Don't ever pooh-pooh the idea of a shampoo and set as having gone out with the ark. It may not be the bread-and-butter work of the majority of salons any more, but it still plays a vital part in hair styling. Many models you see adorning glossy magazines have had their hair set with heated curlers, and long, dressed-up hair has almost certainly been set first. No matter what other fashion styling techniques come and go, setting will remain the classical way of achieving versatility with hair. Permed or curly hair, for instance, can be smoothed out if set on rollers. A growing-out fringe can be disguised if it is set on a number of small rollers for a curly effect or on a few large rollers and swept back off the face.

Before you set your hair, think about the look you want to achieve and choose your roller accordingly. Short hair only needs rollers $\frac{3}{4}$–1 inch in diameter. Bigger rollers can be used on longer hair, but you will still need a supply of the smaller size to wind up the shorter lengths of hair at the nape of the neck and temples. Don't use rollers which are spiked as this will tear and split the hair. For similar reasons, use roller pins which don't have sharp points. A supply of folded paper tissues will be helpful to tuck over the ends of very short hair and give it a smooth line. Pick up small sections of hair at a time – too large a chunk will only make the roller fall out – and if the ends are uneven, wrap

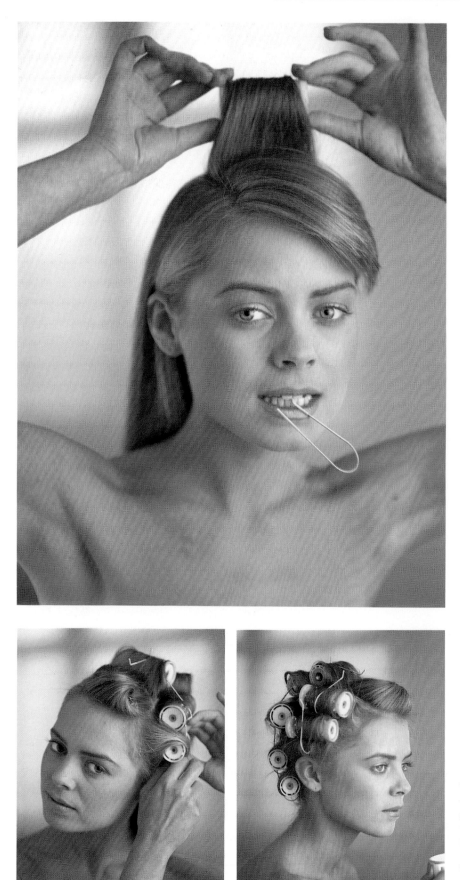

them in a folded paper tissue to make sure they lie flat. Hold the section to be rolled out from the head at a 45° angle and *slowly* and evenly roll it up. You will probably need larger-sized rollers on the top and crown areas of your head, working down to smaller ones along the sides and back. Back and side rollers should generally be wound in the direction that the hair grows.

Once the whole head is wound up, the hair has to be absolutely bone dry before the rollers are removed. Test before unwinding by removing one curl from the thickest part of your hair and feeling between your fingers for dampness. Then wait a few minutes before removing the rollers and brushing the hair through.

Another variation on roller setting, and one which is used in perming, are the soft, bendy rollers which are comfortable to wear and achieve more of a Pre-Raphaelite look. There are several brands available which can be bought from hairdressing salons, chemists and department stores. They are colourful and fun to wear and, because they are soft and comfortable, are ideal for sleeping in if you want a special-occasion style for the next day. These rollers do achieve best effects on longer hair, and if you want to experiment before investing in any, try twist setting to achieve similar results – remember grannie setting her hair in rags? You will need some large tissues or equal-sized pieces of fabric rolled into long tubes. After washing and drying your hair, still leaving it slightly damp, divide off one fairly

These pictures from Vitapointe show the basic hair rolling methods, which apply equally when rolling from wet or when using heated rollers. **Above left:** Hold the section of hair to be rolled at an angle of 45 degrees and then slowly and evenly roll. **Far left:** As a general rule, you'll need larger rollers on the top of the head and the crown areas. **Left:** Always test before unwinding rollers by removing one curl from the thickest part of your hair.

large section. Holding the hair at the ends, twist it along its whole length right up to the roots. Wind the twisted section around the paper or fabric and then tie the two ends together to secure your hair. Just continue like this over the rest of the head and wait with bated breath to see the pretty effect next morning.

Right and below: Modern, bendy rollers are a soft, comfortable and colourful way of achieving a curly look, and there are several types available which can be bought from hairdressing salons or department stores. These pictures from the Molton Brown Hairdressing salon in London show how bendy rollers can make it fun to create a fashionable style.

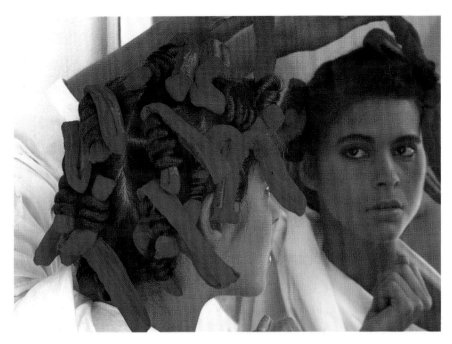

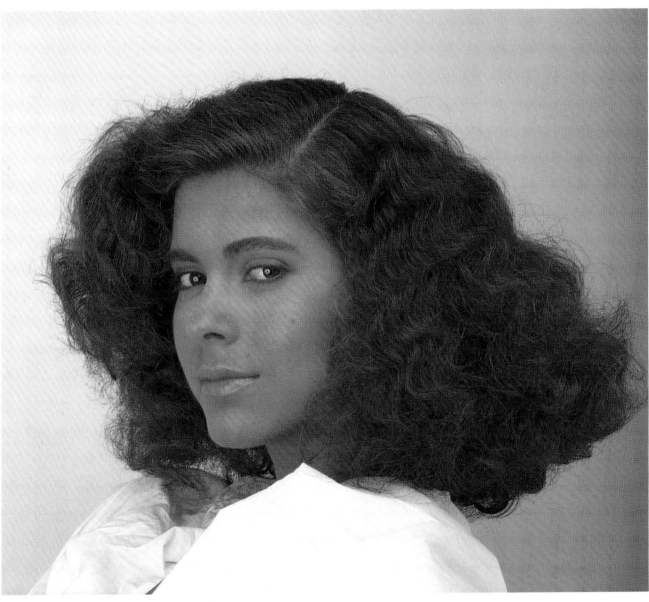

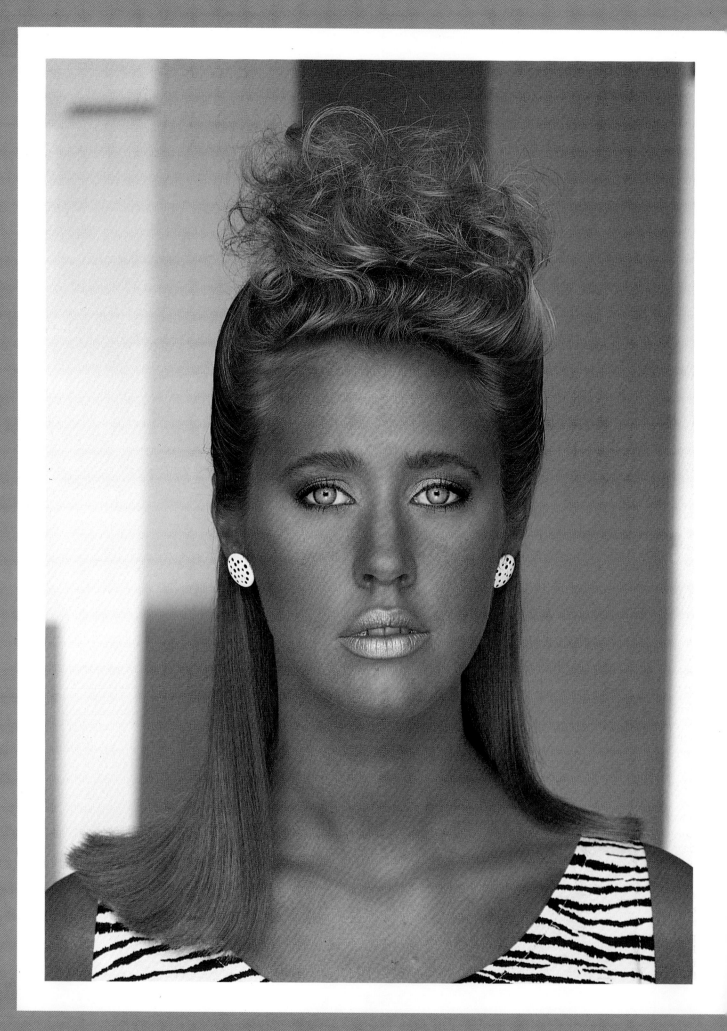

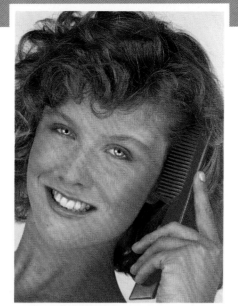

Tools of the trade

Of all the hairdressing paraphernalia we are ever likely to use, brushes and combs remain the fundamental tools of the trade. A hairdresser is never seen without his scissors or tail-comb; and no matter how extravagant or extraordinary a hairstyle may be, at times we are bound to want to touch it up or smooth it into place with a brush or a comb.

Because these instruments are used so frequently, it is important to choose the right ones. A basic rule is never to buy cheap equipment: you simply cannot cut corners where your hair is concerned. Your choice of brush will be very much dictated by the hairstyle you wear but, whatever you select, make sure the brush is heat resistant. Hairdressers can relate horror stories of clients rushing in to have their hair cut off because a brush has melted and tangled the hair beyond redemption under the heat of a hairdryer.

Opposite: Even very straight hair can be given a lift. The front section of the hair was curled with tongs and then pinned on top. **Above:** The Molton Brown Salon in London used their soft, bendy rollers and a wide-toothed comb for this effect.

Fingers were the earliest combs, and were superseded by fish bones fastened between pieces of wood. Greek and Roman women used wood and ivory combs with a double row of teeth, similar to today's fine-toothed combs, for cleaning their heads. Lead combs were used at one time to brighten the hair. The jewellers of the Middle Ages and later devoted their art to the decoration of the double-toothed comb used by the women of the nobility at that time, and examples of these can still be seen in museums today. You will probably need two combs on your beauty check-list: a wide-toothed comb for smoothing and de-tangling hair when wet (wet hair should always be combed, never brushed), and a tail-comb for styling. Hard nylon is the best material but check that the points aren't too sharp. If they are they will tear and damage your hair – that's why hairdressers reel back in horror at the sight of metal combs!

The same applies to brushes. Before you buy, check the bristles by pushing them down into the palm of your hand. You will soon be able to feel whether they are too sharp or not! There are a number of round styling brushes available for blow-drying, and the one you choose depends on your style and required size of curl – the tighter the curl, the smaller the brush. You will also need a good, all-purpose brush for general grooming. Natural bristle brushes are good for fine or delicate hair because they are softer and have rounded ends which won't damage the scalp or hair. That makes them especially good for very long hair too. Nylon and bristle combined can be used for most other hair types, as the firmness of the nylon helps to increase the blood circulation to the scalp while the bristle has a gentle brushing action on the hair.

The correct way to brush your hair is to start from the forehead through to the ends, then bend forward and brush from the nape through the entire length of hair. Make lifting strokes away from the scalp. If the hair is tangled, divide it into sections and gently work your way through until each section is tangle-free. Then throw your head back and gently smooth over the hair.

Always keep your brushes and combs scrupulously clean. Wash them in mild soapy water whenever you shampoo your hair, and leave them to dry at room temperature — never over a radiator or with a hairdryer.

Excessive manipulation of the hair, and that includes brushing, can irritate your scalp and contribute to hair breakage and split ends. It can also cause premature loss of hairs that are in the hair follicle. Just brush your hair as often as is needed to keep it looking neat and attractive.

Hairdryers

So compact and space-age do some hand-held dryers seem these days that we wonder how we ever did without them. They are no longer the cumbersome gadgets we once used to wrestle with and they are a boon for the travelling girl, as many of them fit so neatly into an overnight bag. Today's hairdryers really do help styling hair to be a labour of love rather than a chore, but they can still hinder rather than help a style if they are not used properly. Don't make the common mistake of using too much heat too close to the head too soon. If the hair is dried too quickly your style will just collapse. Rough-dry the roots first, and then concentrate on styling the ends. Always keep the dryer a good distance away from the hair, at least six inches, and use one of the nozzle attachments which should accompany your dryer to control the flow of the heat.

On average, hand-held dryers operate at higher temperatures than hooded dryers so that they can achieve styling effects in a short time. As you are constantly moving the dryer over the head — or should be — the chances of your hair becoming overheated are slight. You will certainly be able to feel the burn on your skin if the setting is too hot!

Good hair care requires gentle handling of hair at all times, and this rule applies even more strongly when hair is being dried.

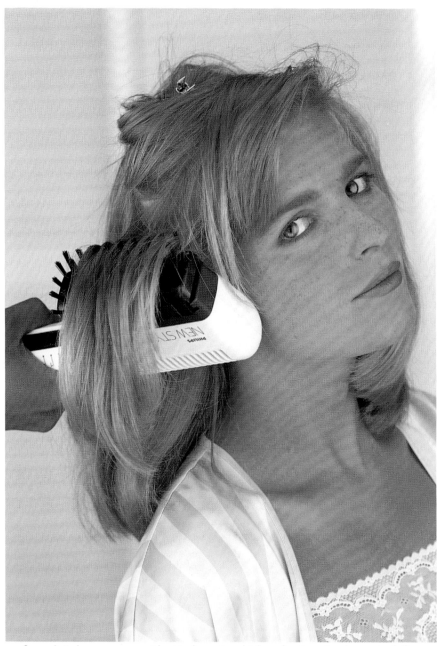

Some hairdryers come with attachments which make it easier to control the direction of the heat. This style is being blow-dried under for a really sleek look (picture courtesy of Philips and *Hair Flair* magazine).

Any rise in temperature softens hair and makes it weaker and more plastic. Damage to hair can easily occur from improper and over-enthusiastic manipulation of the hair while it is hot.

Your choice of dryer is up to you. Apart from size and colour, there are many on the market which have been designed for particularly high-speed drying or to combat the noise problem. Most come with two heat/speed settings — use the higher one for

quickly removing excess moisture and the lower one for styling.

Heated rollers

Hairdressers who regularly style hair for photographic sessions carry their heated rollers around like Bibles. Without doubt they have their place in today's modern styling methods but they should be used with care. Use rollers sparingly, particularly if your hair is dry. It is not a good idea to make any kind of electrical styling aid an everyday habit. Use a protective conditioner or styling mousse beforehand, or look out for flock-covered heated rollers. Alternatively, you could cover them with thin sheets of foam to lessen possible damage from the spikes tearing your hair when you remove them.

For a tighter curl, use the minimum amount of hair on each roller and keep it in longer. To add body rather than curl, use large rollers and brush out vigorously. For best results, always let the curl spring back after taking the roller out and allow the hair to cool before styling.

Styling wands and tongs

It is easy to be deceived by glamorous advertisements showing girls pulling off the motorway and using the rear-view mirror to touch up their hairstyle with a hot brush or comb. Like any other appliance, they have their place, but that place is not necessarily in the glove-box of a Ferrari! Once again, don't let yourself get into the habit of relying on them too regularly as this could have a damaging, drying effect. If you do need to resort to them too frequently, you are either due for a trim to restore the shape to your style or else it needs a total rethink!

Heated brushes and tongs are no longer the cumbersome objects they once were. Thermal curling was originally called 'Marceling' or 'Marcel Waving'. It was named after Marcel Grateau, a Frenchman who perfected the technique in 1875. The original thermal irons, Marcel Irons, had to be made of fine quality steel so that they could be heated evenly. Today, wands and tongs come in two basically different varieties, the attachment types which clip

into the end of the hairdryer, and the independently heated ones. The advantage of the ones that can be attached to a hairdryer is that the heat/speed setting can be controlled. This means that it is possible to put the blower on the cool position, which is kinder to hair.

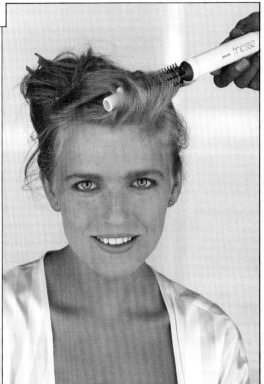

Right and below: For a slightly more ruffled look, a hot styling brush can be put to use on hair which has already been dried. The end result is a sleek style with a little more fullness and body (picture courtesy of Philips and *Hair Flair* magazine).

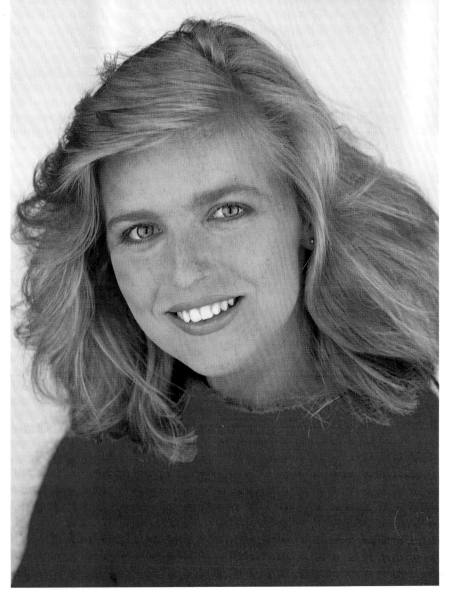

The independent kind — and many now work on butane gas so you don't even need an electric point — are controlled thermostatically, so they shouldn't burn your hair or skin. Whether you want to add soft bouncy waves or smooth out the curl in wavy hair, these appliances are useful when it comes to efficient styling — and they are designed for just that, styling, rather than drying.

Last, but by no means least, a few simple rules to observe when using any electrical styling appliance.

1 Always unplug it from the mains when not in use.

2 Do not wrap the cable around the appliance.

3 Do not place the appliance on any soft material while it is switched on or still hot.

4 Do not take it into the bathroom or use near water.

5 Never leave tongs, brushes or curlers in the hair longer than is necessary.

6 At all times, handle all appliances with care. Your hair is in no one's hands but your own.

This page and opposite: It wouldn't be too difficult to transform a sleek and sporty style like the one above to a head of tumbling, face-framing curls like the one opposite. All you need is practice with the hot curling tongs. Tongs are an absolute boon when it comes to a hair pick-me-up, but remember that they should be just that, and that you shouldn't have to rely on them on a daily basis (pictures courtesy of Philips and *Hair Flair* magazine).

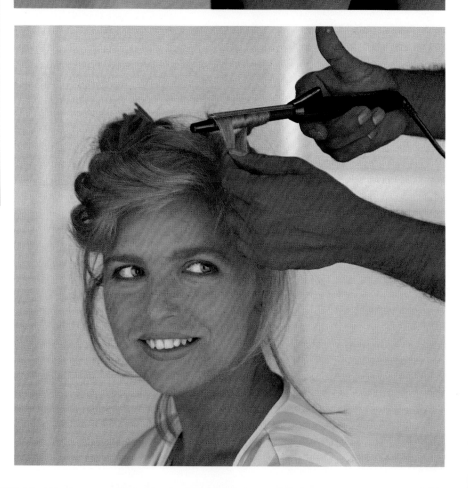

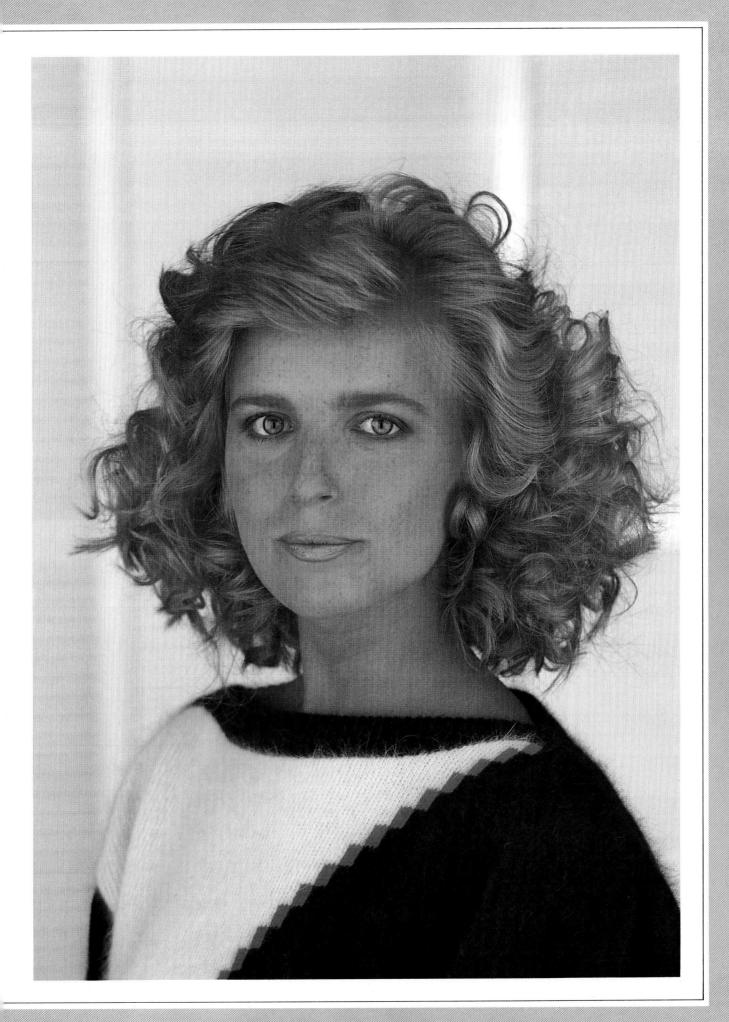

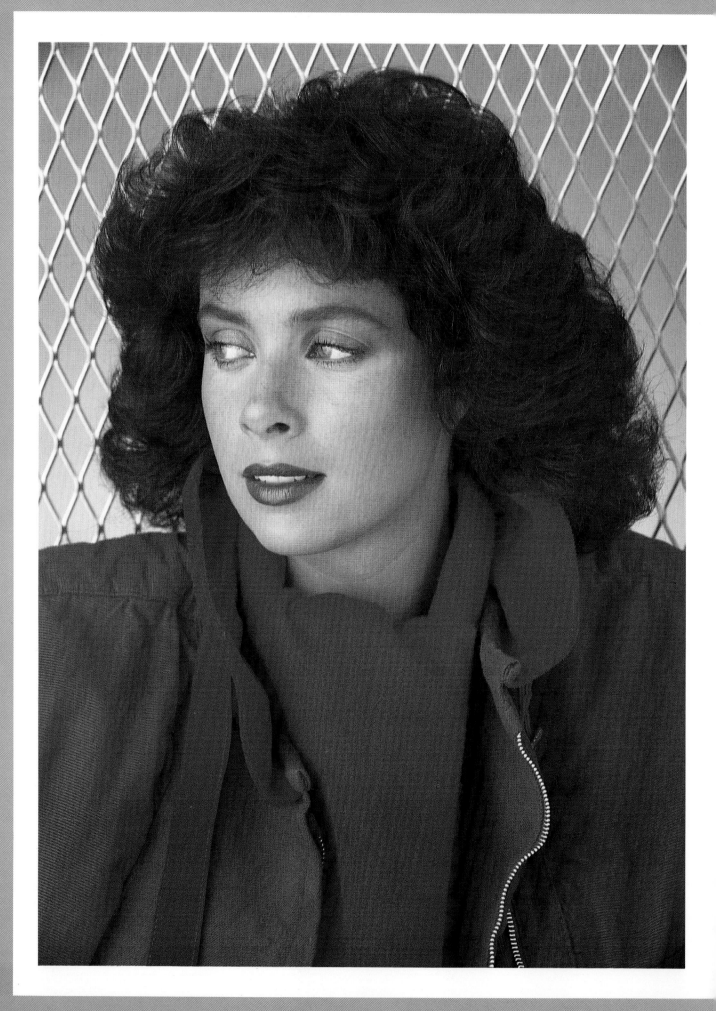

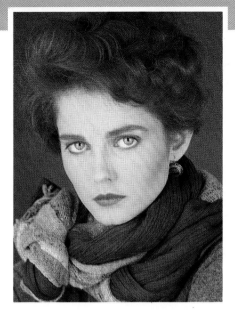

To curl or not to curl

We are, none of us, ever happy with the looks we were born with, but since in most cases our appearance was determined within the womb, there is very little we can do to change things. Although genetics decide whether our hair is straight or wavy, or thick or fine, we have for some time been able to change its structure with chemical treatments. Curls, except to those who are naturally endowed with them, are always desirable. They are pretty, soft and fun and can enhance a style and make hair easier to live with. People have been attempting to put permanent curls in their hair since the time of the Ancient Egyptians and Romans, but on the whole not very successfully. It was not until the 20th century, within about a 30-year period beginning in 1905, that three professional permanent wave methods were introduced.

Perming is nothing new—even the Ancient Egyptians attempted it! But it is a very quick and efficient way of changing the structure of hair.
Opposite: A medium-length head of hair, layered and lightly permed (picture courtesy of Schwarzkopf).
Above: A soft perm from the Molton Brown Hairdressing Salon in London.

The machine permanent method, used in 1905, required electricity to heat large metal clamps which were placed over the client's hair. The hair was wound on the rods from the ends to the head. The machine had long flexible wires attached directly to the large clamps, which were clipped over the rod wound on the client's head. As you can imagine, this was not a very efficient way to curl hair because it required so much equipment.

From the machine permanent came the spin-off preheat permanent wave in 1931. This method eliminated the need for long electrical wires between the machine and the client. Instead, the large clamps were heated on a machine *before* they were placed on the rod wound on the client's head.

It was the machineless permanent wave, however, which removed the use of electricity from the waving process. Instead, it used chemical pads which heated up when moistened with water. After the pad was moistened, it was placed over the rod and held there by a large clamp. This method produced a curl pattern which was 'pressed into the hair' by steam heat from the chemical pads.

All three methods used two main physical principles to curl the hair: winding it tightly around the rod and applying extreme heat. It was in 1940 that the hair waving industry was completely changed – by the introduction of the cold wave. This method employed chemicals, instead of heat, to curl the hair and is still in use today; however, we have since seen even greater developments including the exothermic perm, which has its own heat built in, and this method is as popular with hairdressers as the revolutionary cold wave.

Perming actually changes the structure of the hair and re-forms it to give the desired effect. So if your hair is straight, a perm will curl it according to the size or type of perming rod used. It's important to remember that perming is a very delicate operation, despite all of the improvements in the process and the chemicals used. Home perming lotions are pretty much the same as you would get in a salon – they have to be, or they wouldn't work – but if you are thinking about doing a perm at home, do remember that there are a number of external influences which could possibly affect the end result.

Hairdressers will always warn you off undertaking any kind of chemical treatment at home, not just because they want your trade for themselves but because, unless you are fastidiously careful, they can be a recipe for disaster – a disaster which, more often than not, a hairdresser will have to correct.

When a perm lotion is applied, the hydrogen in it breaks the sulphur bonds in the hair – the ones which maintain its shape – so that it can be reshaped as desired around the perm rod. What locks in this newly formed curl is the neutralizer, the crucial part of the perming process. The oxygen in the neutralizer joins with the hydrogen in the perm lotion to form H_2O – water. That's why your hair seems to drip so much when you have a perm! The neutralizer joins the bond back together by hardening and shrinking the hair shaft and stopping the action of the waving lotion. It's the size of the perm rod which determines the volume of curl, *not* the strength of the perm lotion. Some people leave home perms on for longer than necessary to 'make sure' they take effect. In fact, leaving the perm on for longer doesn't make any difference to the end result at all, and after a while the process will start to reverse itself, leaving the hair nothing short of frizzy.

Perms today are as fashion-orientated as shampoos. They are no longer the painstaking, time-consuming process they used to be and neither will they put us out of pocket. Many perms are designed with client appeal in mind – they may be more attractive or comfortable to wear on the head – but that doesn't mean that the end result will be any better than the more traditional cold wave or exothermic perm. Exothermic perms usually have a lower pH than cold waves and so are kinder

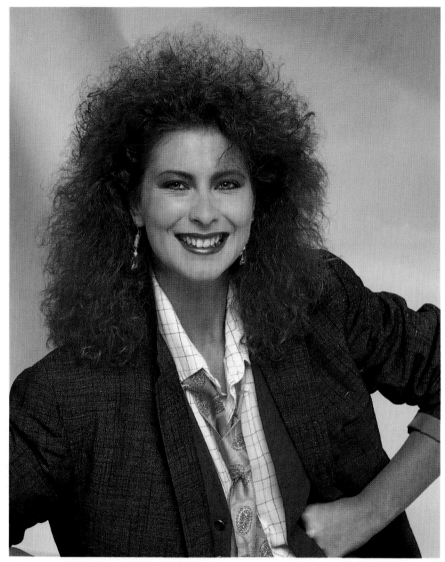

Perming techniques have really come a long way since they were first properly developed at the turn of the century. These sensational curls were created by David Bell of the Mane Street Salon in Bournemouth for Alberto TRESemme/Indola with the help of a self-timing self-heating exothermic perm.

to hair which might be slightly damaged already. If the hair is strong and coarse, however, it will probably need a cold wave to tackle it adequately.

Only a few years ago it was taboo for a hairdresser to think of perming colour-treated hair, but chemical products have developed to such an extent that even that is possible, although a hairdresser will still probably refuse to perm heavily bleached hair. He doesn't want a client with hair that resembles nothing more than soggy cotton wool. It's important that before having a perm you are completely honest with your

hairdresser about anything you might have put on your hair yourself. If you have applied peroxide or metallic dyes at home it could have a disastrous effect on your hair and it's no good complaining when it's too late.

So far we have only pointed out the pitfalls of perming, but perms can do a lot to improve the look and condition of your hair. They can be used to achieve a shaggy look, tight curls, loose waves or simply to add body and, if your hair is very greasy or lank, they will have a slight drying effect which could mean less washing and more manageability.

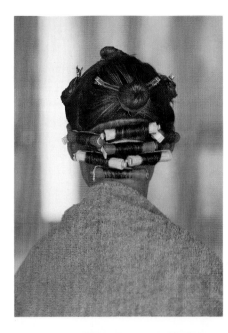 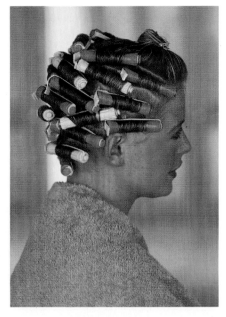 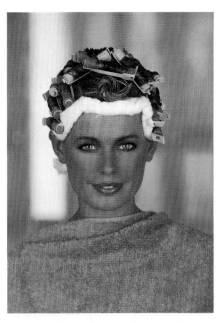

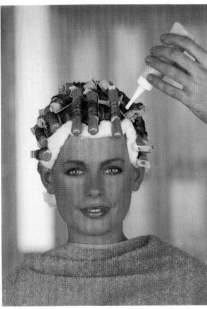

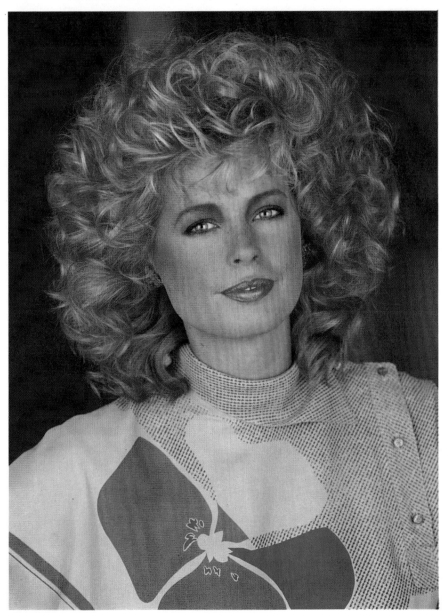

This style was created by Bastian for Alberto TRESemme/Indola.

Top: The hair is permed using a brick-work winding technique with medium and large rods taken at random sections.

Centre: The side and back sections are wound directionally towards the back of the head using alternate rod sizes, while the front and side sections are wound directionally forward.

Top right: Here you can see the crown section which has been wound directionally forward in a brick-work fashion. Cotton wool was placed around the hairline before the fringe section was wound.

Main picture: Once the perming process time is up and the perm properly finished, the hair is dried under a lamp and each curl carefully brushed through.

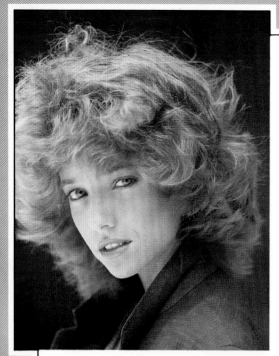

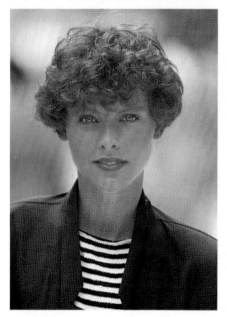

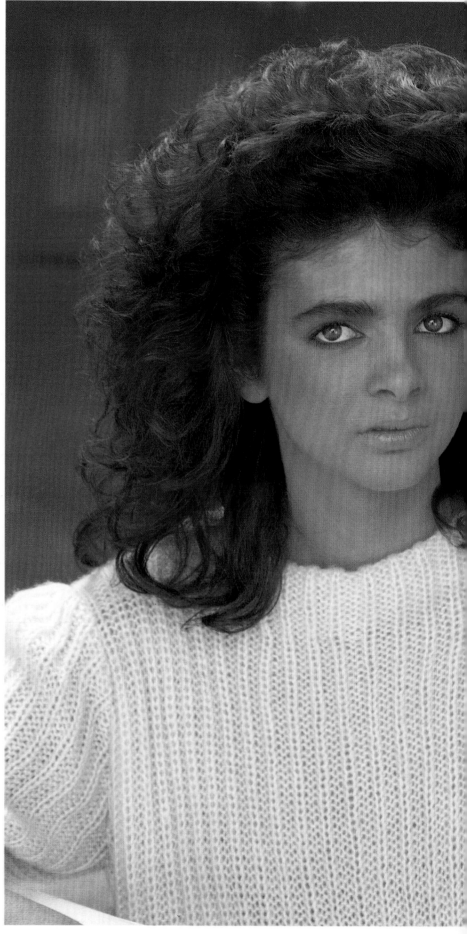

The photographs on these pages show just how versatile a perm can be.

Top: A mid-length layered style from Glemby International lightly permed to achieve a casual, tousled effect.

Above: Very short haircuts, like this one from Glemby International, can still be successfully permed and the soft curls help eliminate what might otherwise be harsh lines.

Main picture: Shoulder-length permed hair can be styled to suit any occasion (hair by the Taylor Ferguson Salon, Glasgow).

Opposite top: A gentle perm used by Schwarzkopf in this picture to add body to the hair.

Opposite bottom: Another lightly permed head of hair from Schwarzkopf. This one could easily be made to look a bit more unruly with the help of a little mousse and the scrunch drying technique.

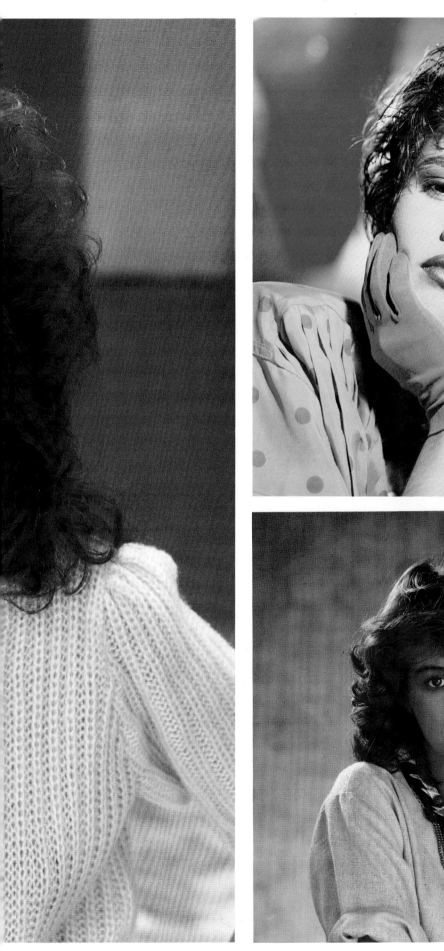
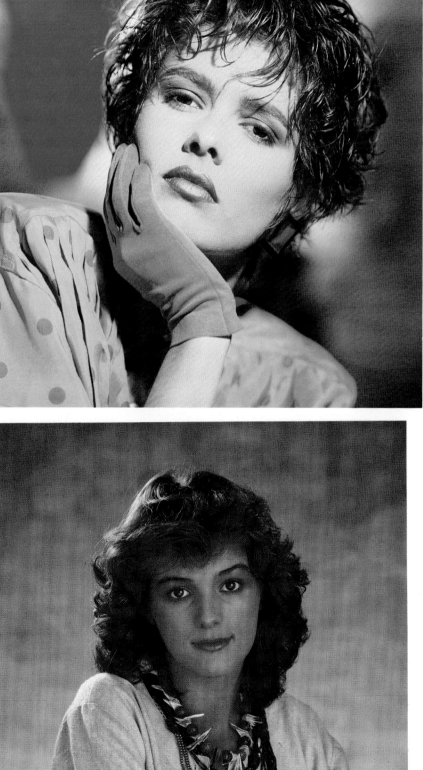

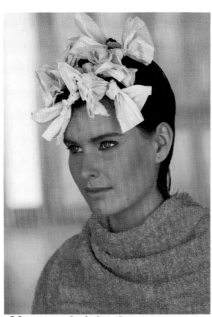

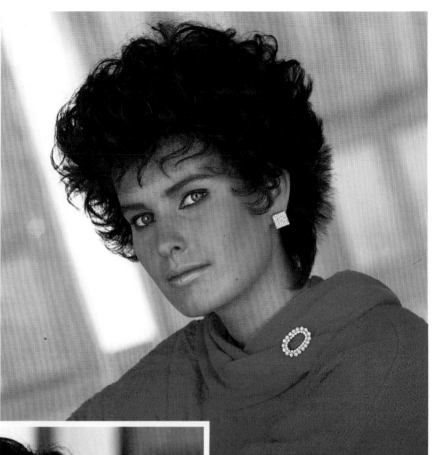

Above and right: Bastian created this style for Alberto TRESemme/Indola by perming it on top, using tissue paper to give it volume. The tissues were rolled into a cylindrical shape and one-inch sections of the hair wound around the tissues, which were then knotted.

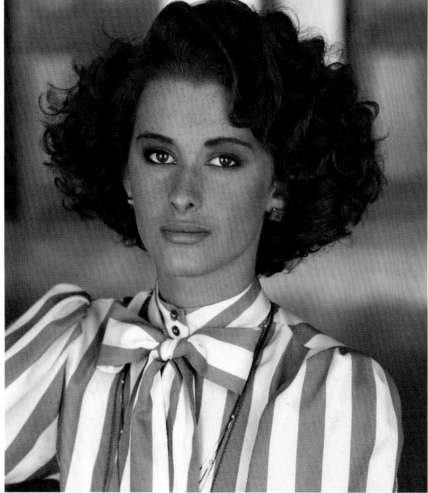

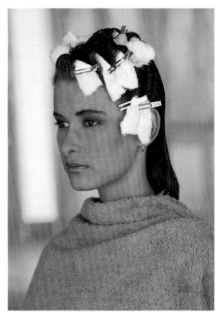

Above and left: The first section of hair at the forehead was wound around cotton wool towards the crown and secured. The second section was wound towards the forehead and the technique continued to the crown (hair by Bastian for Alberto TRESemme/Indola).

Techniques

There are several kinds of perming technique used by hairdressers to achieve different effects.

Demi waves are a kind of perm rather than a technique. They are slightly weaker than normal perms and don't break down so many bonds. The effect is a bend or 'lift' to the hair which will last about six weeks.

Root perming is another way of giving hair a lift without curl. Cling-film is usually placed on the ends of the hair to protect it and it is only the root area of the hair that is treated. Root perms are really best for short hair, or for hair which has a perm growing out because, as the hair grows, the perm will fall to the middle of the hair and the roots will appear flat.

An end perm is when the hair is just curled at the bottom. It is mainly used on long hair or on a style such as a one-length bob, where it is desirable to bend the ends in to keep them under.

Weave perming is truly versatile. It involves perming some sections of the hair and leaving the rest unpermed, creating a natural, textured effect.

Spiral winding is a method of winding the hair on to the perming rods, designed like corkscrews, to produce Pre-Raphaelite waves on longer hair.

Watch the products you use on your hair after a perm. What suited it before may not be quite so beneficial now, and you may find that you will have to change your shampoo or conditioner, or both. An intensive conditioning treatment is always a good idea after a perm, and then on a regular basis, but you should already be looking after your hair with this much consideration!

Perming pitfalls

Perming, then, can do a lot to enhance your looks and con-

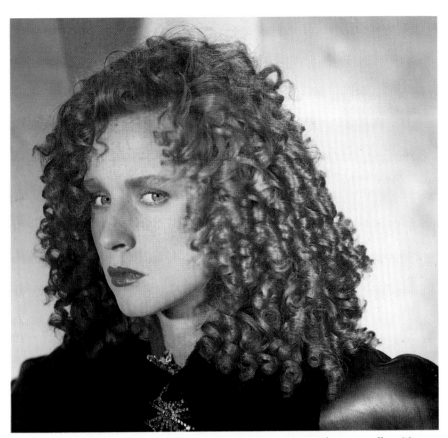

Perms can create a hint of softness and volume or a more dramatic effect like this one from Schwarzkopf; a spiral perm produces masses of corkscrew curls.

fidence, and if you have always yearned for a perm but never quite had the courage, then go ahead and try. It's almost a foregone conclusion that you will be delighted with the result. But perming is a process which *can* go wrong and it's important that you are aware of some of the problems which can occur, so that you aren't too tempted to experiment casually at home.

Some hairdressers are still sceptical about perming hair during pregnancy, although there is no real evidence to support their doubts. Their main worry is that because of the hormonal changes in the body at this time, a perm might not 'take' so well. But in a normal healthy woman, there should be no difference in the ability of the hair to curl. After all, just as at any other time, the hair which is visible during pregnancy is dead and therefore not subject to physiological alteration. It can only be changed by external treatments – such as bleaches,

waving or hair straighteners. The new hair which grows during the nine months of pregnancy is that which is closest to the scalp and so is least affected by the permanent waving process anyway. Perming is not a good idea if you are about to go on holiday. The lure of easier-to-manage hair is an attractive one, but you should weigh against that the possibility of untold damage from the climate of a hot holiday resort, and it really is more sensible to wait until you get home. If you swim regularly in a pool it is best not to have a perm at all. The chlorine in pool water is very damaging to hair and, together with a perm, will ruin it.

If you want colour and a perm, it is always best to have the perm done first. This is because when hair is coloured, particularly with woven highlights, there are many different textures in your hair – yet the same perm lotion has to be used all over. It is much better, therefore, to perm a head which has the same hair type through-

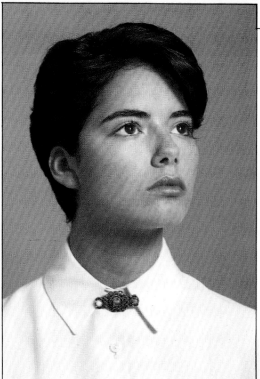

out. Remember, too, that the neutralizer in a perm does affect the hair's natural colour, particularly when it is light brown, so it's often even a good idea to have colour added afterwards.

Perms can go wrong for several reasons and the most obvious is that the lotion wasn't applied evenly. Something which happens more frequently is that a client

Left and below: This before-and-after from Schwarzkopf shows how perms can be used to add elegance to a flat, simple style. A perm is also a very good way of growing out short hair.

could be sitting in a draught – particularly likely in the summer, when a hot salon may have its windows and doors open. The side which is more insulated will take more quickly than the side affected by the draught, which will therefore be looser. Imagine how that can affect a home perm, when you are likely to get up and wander around from one temperature to another, if only to answer the telephone, which may be in a draughty hallway near the front door. This is why hairdressers often prefer an exothermic perm, which is a kind of safety precaution as it has its own built-in heat. If you are at all worried about this happening – and hairdressers are usually professional enough to guard against it – then look for a salon which has a separate draught-proof perming and tinting area away from the main styling floor.

The rinsing and neutralizing stages of perming have got to be done thoroughly and not too quickly. If a perm rod isn't rinsed enough, the neutralizer won't work properly. If a perm appears to go straight at the back, near the nape of the neck, it's because that area, when placed in the backwash, has been neglected during the rinsing process. In many salons it is the junior who carries out this task and he or she may not realize how important a procedure it is. If you have any reason to believe that it is not being done properly, ask relevant but tactful questions about the perm and how it varies from others in order to make the junior think about whether or not they are obeying the manufacturer's instructions to the letter.

Don't be daunted by the pros and cons of perming. It can be an excellent body builder and morale booster, as long as you remember – handle with care.

Opposite: A well-conditioned permed head from the Molton Brown Hairdressing Salon, London.

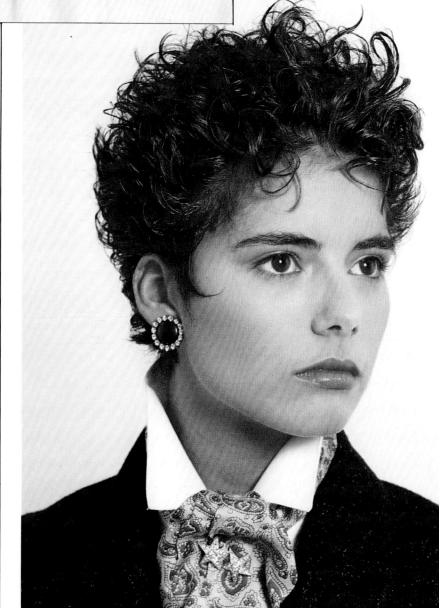

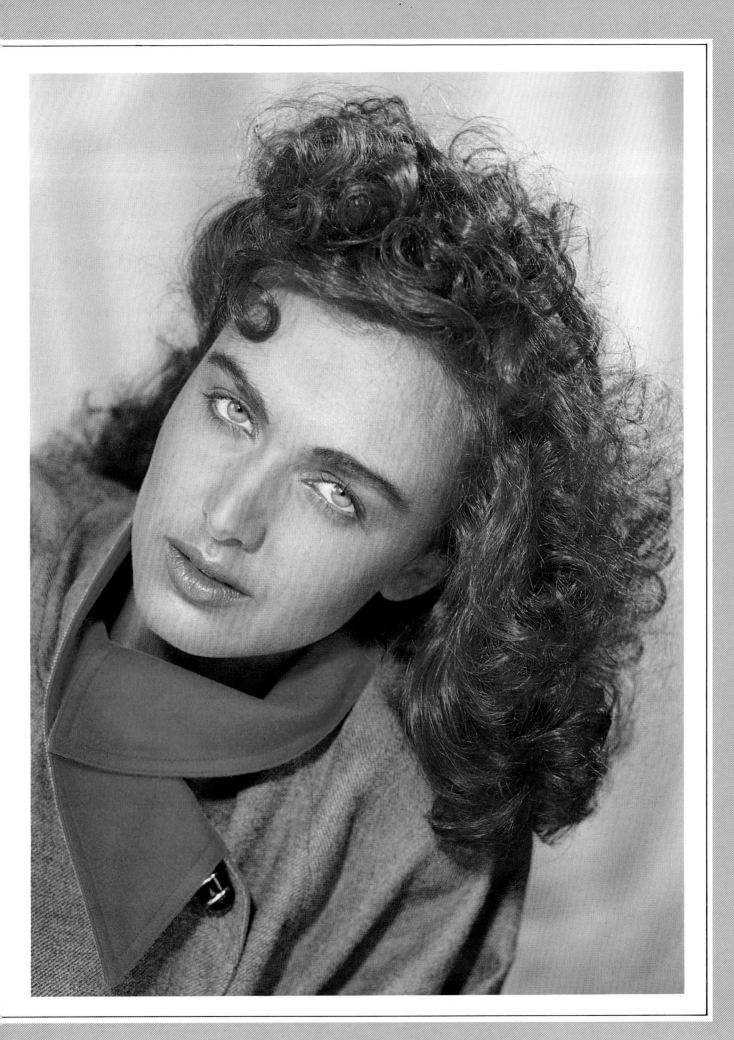

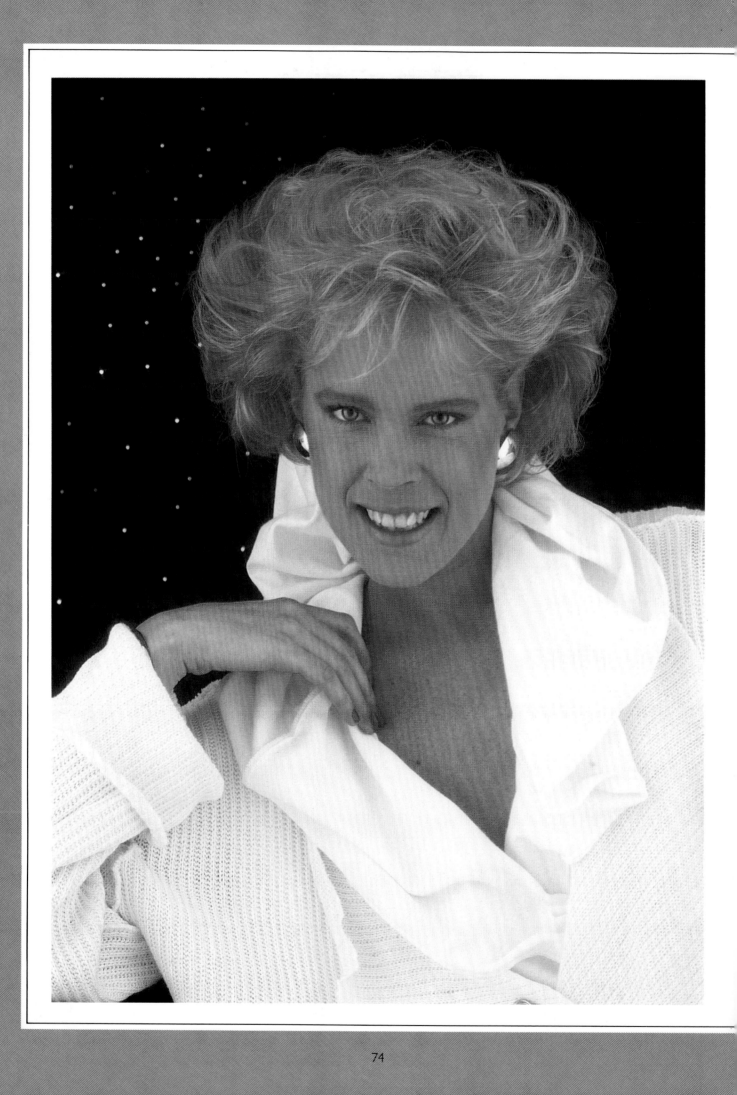

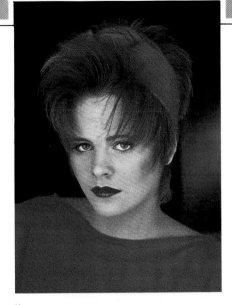

Colour up

In these days of high-technology hairdressing, exhibitionism and overwhelming creativity hair colour doesn't just stop with the hues of the rainbow. No matter what your hairstyle, type or natural shade, a touch of colour, be it subtle or sensational, is always a pleasing sight. It can even improve the texture and condition of your hair and bring out in you confidence you never knew existed!

The great thing about colouring techniques of the 1980s is that they are no longer the great burden they used to be. Remember those mothers, aunts or family friends who years ago never seemed to be out of the hairdressing salon because their roots constantly needed 'touching up'? With today's vast array of coloured mousses and gels and fun semi-permanent colouring techniques, hair colour isn't anything like the commitment it once was. We can even change the colour of our locks every week if we want

Opposite: Highlights can be used subtly to enhance the hair's natural colour or can create a truly sun-kissed look (*Hair & Beauty* magazine). **Above:** Schwarzkopf had semi-permanent copper highlights applied to this style.

to; and if we prefer to opt for an all-over tint, since fashion dictates that anything goes, it's often perfectly acceptable to let roots grow out naturally.

People have been changing their hair colour for thousands of years, and hair colouring products have been made from a variety of substances. Vegetable dyes were among the earliest kinds of hair colour, and are still used today in more colour-orientated salons. About 4000 years ago Egyptians used henna to redden the hair and camomile to lighten it. Both of these products coat the cuticle, or the outside, of the hair shaft. With each application they build up on the hair to make the colour more intense.

Henna is the reddish dye from the leaves of the lawsonia plant. There are many different types, from different countries, with varying strengths. Henna works best on brown hair, the darker the better – that's why it was such a favourite with the dark-haired Egyptians. Camomile is a plant which grows in Britain in wild and cultivated states. There are various species, not unlike a large daisy. The flower heads can be collected and dried and either left

like that or ground into a powder. The powder can be made into a paste and applied to the hair in the form of a pack which, after about 15 minutes, is washed off. The result will be a golden glint which will vary according to the basic colour of the hair beforehand and the duration of time for which the paste is left on. Rhubarb root is the strongest of the natural lighteners and it will brighten and lift the colour from all hair types. To make an infusion, boil two ounces of rhubarb root in two pints of water, cover and simmer for about an hour. Allow the liquid to cool, and strain it. Use the liquid as a final rinse, running it through your hair several times.

In later years metallic salt dyes came into use. These are a combination of copper, lead, silver and other metals as well as a weak acid. The salts undergo a chemical change to deposit a coloured film along the hair shaft without penetration.

These preparations had several disadvantages. Several applications were often required to make any appreciable change in the colour of the hair and there were a limited number of shades available. The dyes tended to

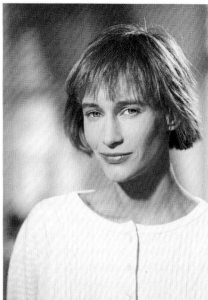

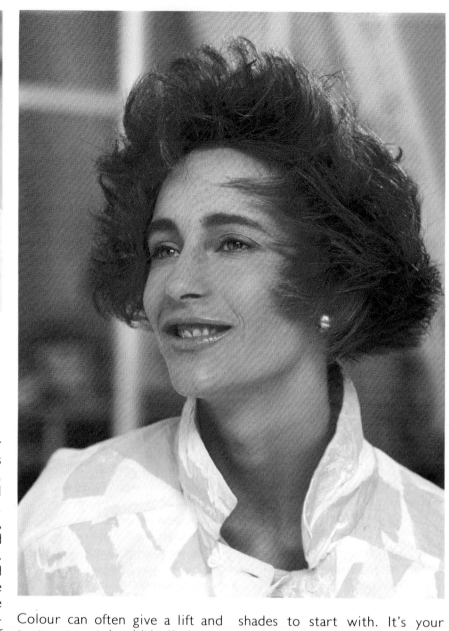

Above and right: Alberto TRESemme/Indola applied three semi-permanent colours to this model's hair to tone down her existing highlights and complement her skin colour. One colour was used all over, and two more applied to the existing highlights to result in a warm, brown-red colour.

produce intense colours rather than the muted, lighter shades which are often more becoming, and the metallic salt dyes could interfere with permanent waving.

Over the years compound dyes, a combination of metallic salt and vegetable dyes, were developed. However, these dyes, too, had serious disadvantages because vegetable and herbal dyes coat the hair too much. Metallic salt preparations can cause discoloration of the hair and compound dyes were responsible for a combination of these problems.

As with perming techniques, colour has now been developed to such an advanced stage that these problems rarely occur. Today, colouring falls into three basic categories – temporary, semi-permanent and permanent. But before we go on to talk about each of these in turn, let's look at a few guidelines to help you know when to colour up and which shades will suit you best. Colour is usually the final stage in the creation of a new hairstyle, and it is best applied after a perm if a perm is necessary.

Colour can often give a lift and texture to a style which eliminates the need for a perm altogether. Think about your colour for a long time – wait at least a week between appointments after having your hair cut so you can consider the kind of colour you would like – and discuss it with your stylist or tinter. Keep an eye open for salons which either specialize in colour or have tinters/permers who do just that. If it's a job a hairdresser does specialize in, he's bound to have the time, patience and inspiration you are looking for. If you are at all doubtful about the end result, then go for temporary or semi-permanent colours in subtle shades to start with. It's your prerogative to choose something that will enhance your natural hair colour, rather than make a topic of conversation, although colour is a bit like make-up – if you are going to wear it, it's nice to let it show.

The only time to think about saying no to colour is when the condition of your hair is seriously at risk. It is possible for colour to improve the condition of hair because it opens up the cuticles and closes them again, smoothing them out and making the hair shine. But with very dry, porous hair the cuticle is raised along the hair shaft, allowing the colour to penetrate unevenly, and the result will be patchy and dull.

Before choosing a shade, think about your natural skin tone. Warmth can be added to a pale skin with reds, chestnuts and golds, but if you have a ruddy complexion avoid those colours and stick to slightly ashen tones. A very light colour is really too great a contrast to your natural looks if you have darker skin, so select a warm brown or burgundy shade. Remember that if you have a pale complexion and want something dark – and this can work well – your make-up has got to be strong too. You should also make allowances for an extrovert personality being able to wear a more vibrant colour than an introvert one. Bear in mind that as skin ages, it loses its firmness and a certain amount of colour. Older women are therefore not recommended to use very dark hair colours which may be too harsh for their skin tones. Now let's look more closely at some of the hair colouring techniques available.

Temporary colours

These are exactly what they say they are. They remain on the hair only until the next shampoo. They thinly coat the hair cuticle but do not penetrate into the cortex. Temporary colours have, in past years, been available in many shapes and forms – rinses, sprays, creams, powders, crayons and shampoos, some of which have had nothing more than gimmick value.

Rinses are among the most common temporary colours used today. They contain different combinations of chemicals and colours made from vegetables and herbs. The cuticle layer of the hair shaft, the one that protects the cortex, attracts rinses and the colour settles into the crevices of the cuticle and lightly coats it.

Coloured mousses and gels, some with glitter or a metallic sheen for special occasions, are really fun to use and wash out easily. They are available in a spectrum of dazzling colours, as well as more subdued ones, and can even be brushed or combed through the hair for a highlighting effect. You will probably need a lot of practice to become a real expert in the use of coloured gels and mousses, but because they are so readily available and relatively inexpensive, experimenting can be great fun. Be careful, though, if your hair is already very dry, porous or bleached, as these products may need more than one wash before they disappear.

Semi-permanent colours

As the name implies, these are half-way between temporary and permanent colours. They partially penetrate the cortex and put some colour inside the hair. Semi-permanent colours contain chemicals which raise the pH level to an alkaline range of 7–9. This alkalinity causes the cuticle to swell so that some of the colour pigment can enter the cortex. It is the

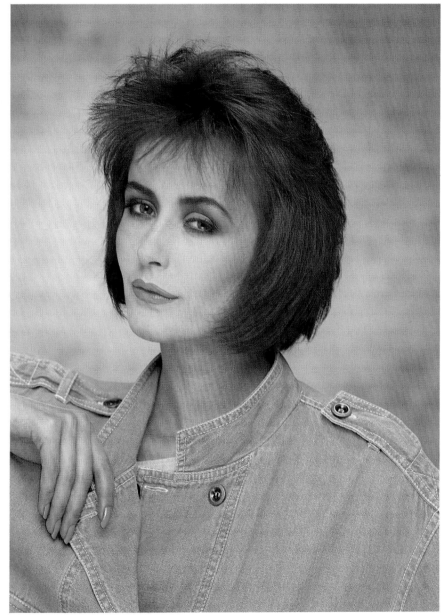

Temporary colours remain on the hair only until the next shampoo and are a good way of experimenting with colour. Schwarzkopf used a Mahogany Red temporary colour on this head of hair.

sulphur molecules which contain the colour pigment and these molecules attach themselves to the keratin (hard protein fibre) of the cuticle and to some of the salt bonds in the cortex. The cuticle is stained and the cortex partially coloured.

Because they do not completely penetrate the cortex, instead of remaining in the hair until it grows (as with permanent colours) they gradually fade out, usually between four and eight shampoos. They can produce immediate or gradual colour change, depending on the method of application, but repeated applications at weekly intervals will deepen the colour to that achieved in the long, single application.

Semi-permanent colours contain no bleaching agents so, like temporary colours, they cannot lighten hair. But they will enrich its natural colour – they are ideal for making mousey hair more interesting – and help tone in early grey hairs. Most semi-permanents also contain conditioners and so will add a nice, natural lustre to the hair.

Permanent colours

These penetrate the cuticle of the hair and deposit colour in the cortex of the shaft. After they have entered the cortex, the coloured molecules of the dye base combine with oxygen from the hydrogen peroxide in the product to make large molecules of dye. These newly formed molecules are too large to pass back through the imbrications, so they are permanently locked within the cortex. The new coloration lasts just as long as the hair does and that is why, when 'new' hair grows, the roots have to be 'touched up'.

Only permanent colours, in the form of lighteners or bleach, can lighten your hair and virtually any form of colour change is possible

Right: The hair is prepared to be treated with a fade-out semi-permanent colour by Alberto TRESemme/Indola.
Below left: The product is applied to the back of the head and the hair roughly sectioned to ensure even coverage.
Bottom left: The colour is massaged thoroughly into the hair until it lathers well.
Below right: The entire head is covered and the colour worked through from the roots to the ends.
Bottom right: Colour is combed through and left for 15 minutes.
Opposite: The hair is rinsed and styled.
Who'd have thought that such a quick and simple salon process could result in such a stunning effect?

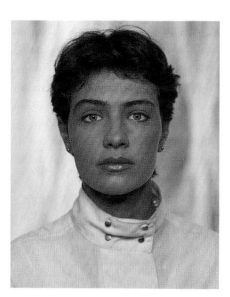

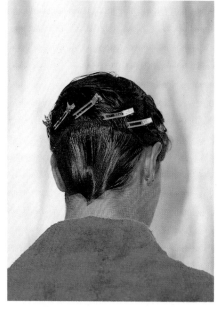

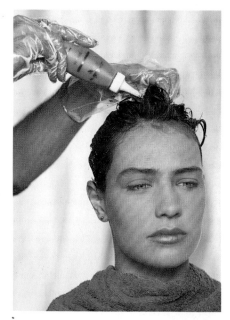

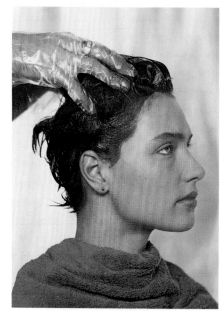

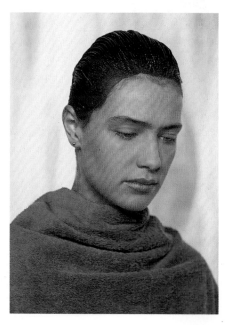

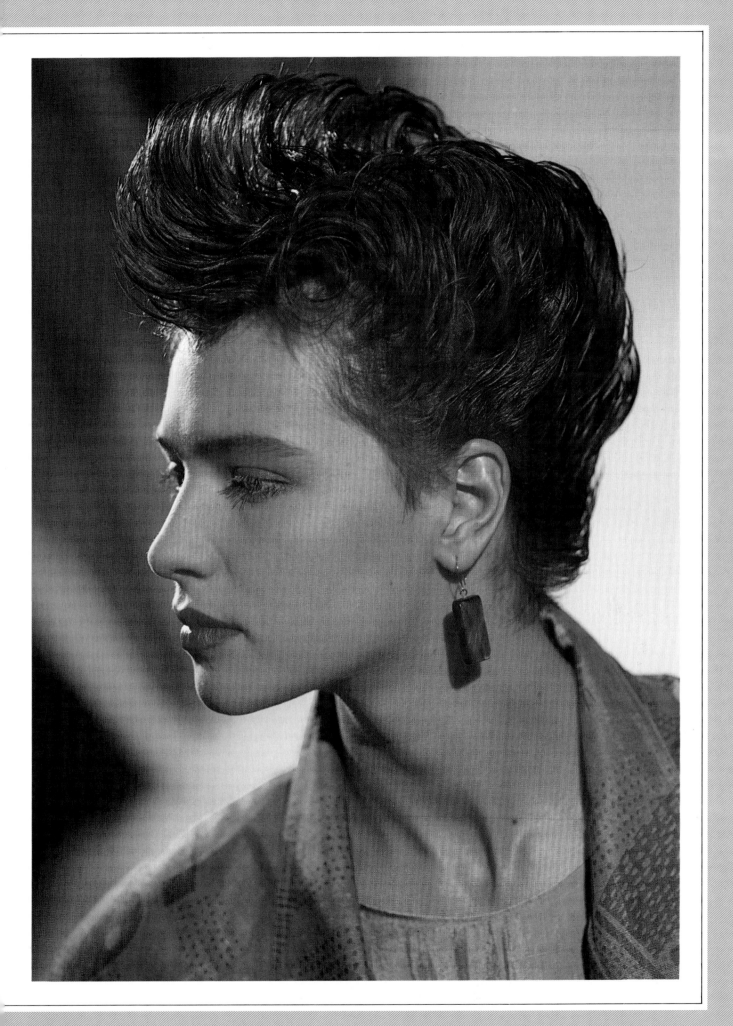

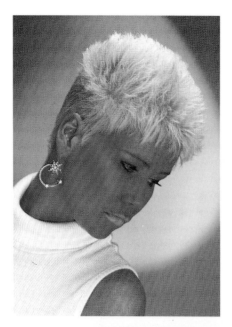

with permanent colours, although most of us wouldn't choose to look too unnatural. Although permanent colour can only grow out, the colour can fade if the cuticle is opened. This is possible through over-use of electrical styling aids or as a result of too much heat from the sun if, for instance, you go on holiday immediately after having an application of permanent colour.

Permanent colours can look as subtle or as severe as you want them to. **Left:** A heavily bleached look from Crimpers in London. **Below:** Schwarzkopf applied a light mocha brown and hazel blond permanent colours to this head to bring out the best in its precision cut.

Years ago excessive bleaching was too easy a trap to fall into. Fashion-conscious females really did think that blondes had more fun and nothing would convince them otherwise. Most salons today value their reputations too highly to bleach a client's hair continually and risk ruining it. If hair is bleached excessively, it may become harsh and strawlike and even break. This damage occurs because peroxide, the bleaching agent, attacks keratin as well as hair colour pigment, causing the hair to lose its elasticity, resilience and tensile strength. The damage is limited to that portion of the hair that is treated, so future hair

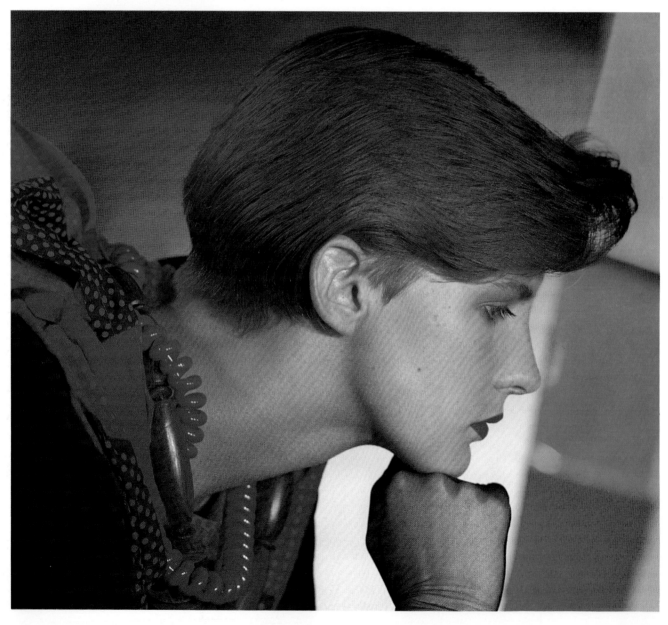

growth is not affected, but that means a long wait before you have a healthy, virgin head of hair again. The great advantage of permanent colour is that if you particularly like a shade and know it is going to suit you, it is more economical than any of the other hair colorants because it lasts longer.

Highlights

Highlights and lowlights are by far the most popular form of colouring in salons. Highlights, as the name implies, lighten the hair. Shades which tone in with, rather than lighten the hair in any way, are called lowlights.

There are numerous advantages with this colouring technique. For you, the client, it's an ideal way of building up colour or subtly enhancing your hair's natural colour without the problem of regrowth. For, although regrowth does occur, as only strands of hair are tinted or bleached, they are not so visible as in complete head tints.

For the hairdresser, partial colouring gives enormous scope for creativity. Highlighting and lowlighting are only the forerunners of partial colouring; there are many other methods which change according to fashion and seasons. Whether bleach or tint is used on your hair depends on the kind of result you are looking for. You might want that after-holiday, bleached-beach-beauty look, or something more delicate, although it is possible to make hair quite light these days just by using tint rather than bleach.

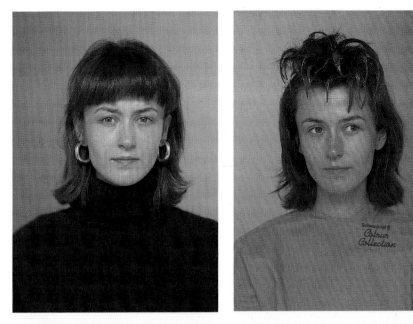

Top left: This style needed lift and interest so Schwarzkopf set to work with its palette of colours. Semi-permanents were used here; they cannot lighten the hair but are ideal for enriching its natural colour, making mousey hair more interesting or for toning in early grey hairs. **Top right:** Schwarzkopf applied its Copper Mahogany semi-permanent colour across the top of the hair. **Right:** The end result is a truly visible difference!

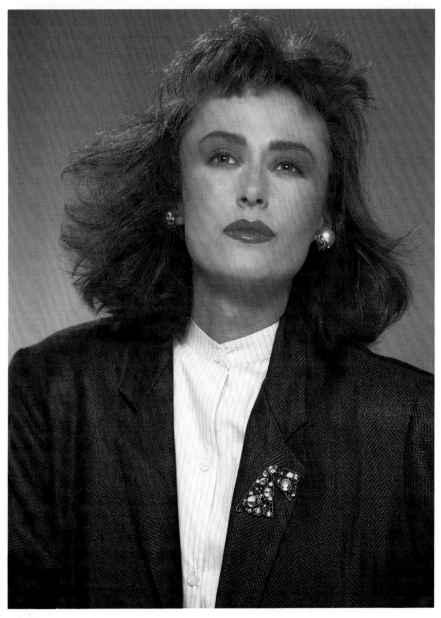

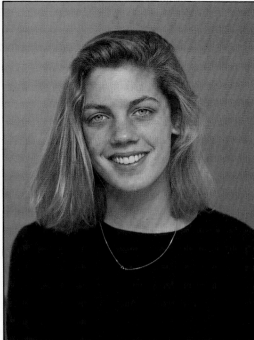

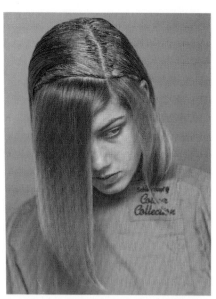

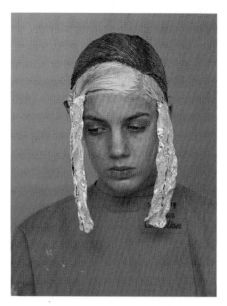

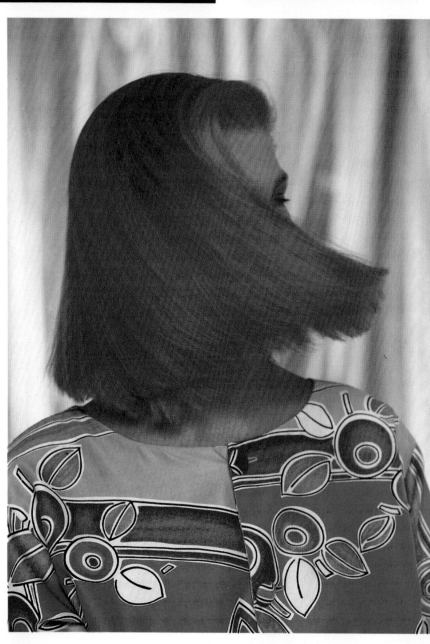

Above: The steps involved in re-colouring hair which needed a lift. Two permanent colours were used from the Schwarzkopf range, including bleach in the front sections to brighten it. A light blond was applied through the back of the hair. The tin foil method used here is said to be kindest to the hair. **Main picture:** The breathtaking result.

The main methods used for highlighting hair are: using tinfoil, a cap, cling-film, or specially manufactured plastic packets. Tinfoil highlights take some considerable time – hours if your hair is very long. Some of the more up-market hairdressing salons will highlight only with tinfoil, as it is said to be kindest to the hair; it is also extremely effective and doesn't tug on the hair strands. However, because of the time required it also makes the appointment a more lucrative one for the salon! Strands of hair are selected, placed on a small square of foil, the bleach or tint is applied and the foil is wrapped around the hair until the process is complete.

The cling-film method works on a similar basis, with the advantage that the stylist – and you – can see what is going on and how the hair is taking. The specially manufactured plastic packets which have been used in salons in the past few years do speed up this process, as they are not as awkward to use as cling-film.

The cap method isn't any less becoming, but it is probably less comfortable than the other methods. A plastic cap is placed on the head, selected strands are pulled through with a hook (this can make the eyes smart) and the product is then applied. Because this method is much less time-consuming for the stylist, it is inevitably the cheapest. Highlights and lowlights can cost anything from £15 to £100 depending on which part of the country you live in, the kind of salon you choose, which method you adopt and how long your hair is. So make sure you see the price list first, or you could be in for a nasty shock, which could sour the pleasure of any hairstyle, no matter how wonderful!

Other partial colouring techniques

Colour is now often applied to suit the hairstyle and that's how some of the numerous partial colouring techniques have been born. Others are created by colouring houses to promote their products through magazines but, for whatever reasons they were created, they provide imaginative food for thought. They certainly illustrate how diverse the world of colour can be.

Tortoise-shelling involves putting three or four colours on to the hair in alternating sections. It works best on brown heads with a colour combination such as red, hazel, honey and blond.

Comb-on colour means just that; colour is combed into the hair after it has been cleaned and styled. This is a good technique for semi-permanent colours in high fashion shades.

Naturalizing is a nice introduction to permanent colouring as it gives a natural look, achieved by picking out and accentuating natural lights in the hair. Two or

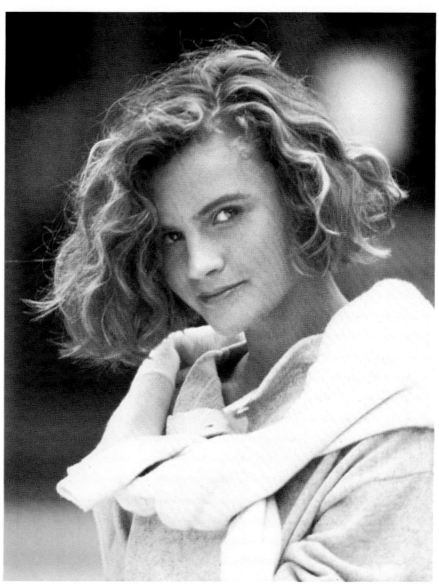

Highlighting needn't be subtle. As this picture from Glemby International shows, it can be used to create more of a streaked effect if the client wants her colour to look more obvious or make a strong colour statement.

three colours are used, but only small sections of the hair are coloured, so there is no problem with regrowth.

Block colouring is good for emphasizing a strong shape, such as a bob, because the colour is applied in large sections. Block colouring lends itself to dramatic effects and it can be used on hair which has already been coloured.

Scrunch colouring is another method suitable for applying semi-permanents in high fashion colours. Colour is applied by hand on to hair which has been cut and dried as if the hair were being scrunch-dried into place.

Touch colouring is where the tips of the hair are lightened to create a sun-kissed effect.

Two-toning has been used if the front section of the hair is coloured a shade lighter than the natural hair colour, and the back a shade darker (or vice versa).

Some of these methods will come and go as quickly as seasons and fashions change; others will become classics. But at least you can see that the sky's the limit where colour is concerned, and there's nothing to stop you asking for one of these techniques, or even inventing an effect of your own.

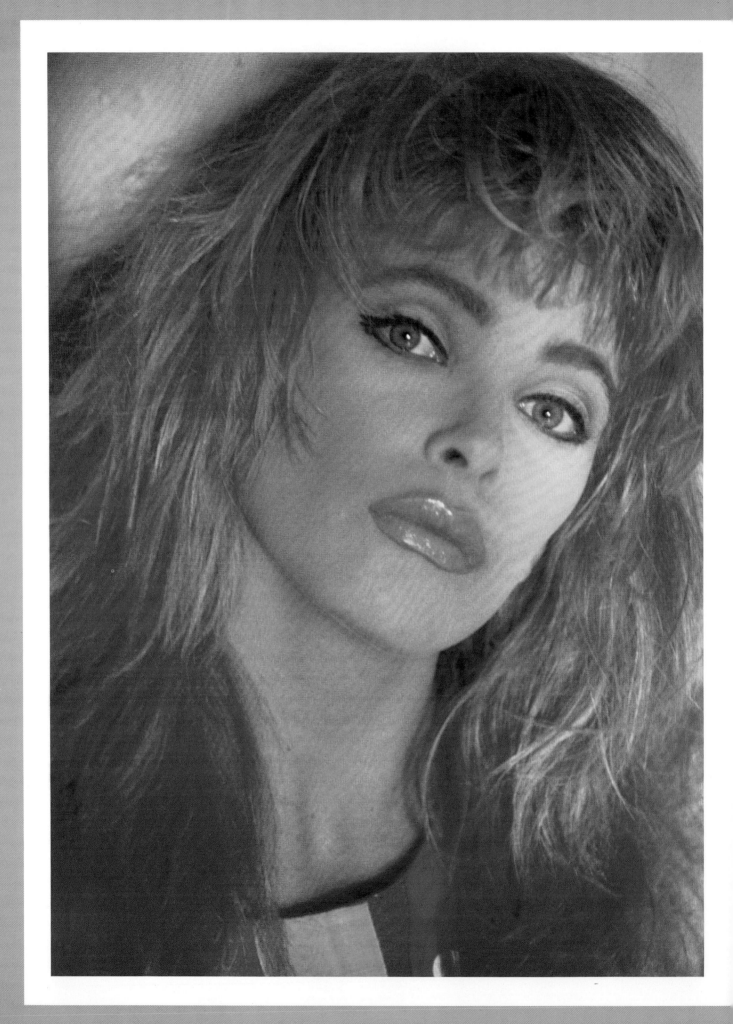

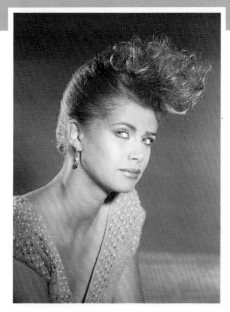

Along different lines

Hair cutting trends come and go as quickly as fashions but, like your favourite pair of old denim jeans, long hair never really goes out of vogue. In the 1960s it slipped temporarily from favour with the advent of mini-skirts and matching hairstyles. Suddenly it was discovered that short, snappy styles could be so much easier to care for, and highly flattering for pert young faces.

There are romantics among us, however, who will always prefer long hair. It is softer, extremely versatile and often very eye-catching. Models are always encouraged to keep their hair at least at shoulder length to enable stylists on photographic sessions to do more with it. This trend appears to be catching on because research carried out by an international hairdressing organization reveals that 30% of women today wear their hair shoulder length or longer.

Long hair takes a lot of work, but the result pays dividends. **Opposite:** Schwarzkopf show how layers can work beautifully on long hair. **Above:** The Stevie Buckle Hair Salon in London have curled the front section of this hair and put up the rest for a sophisticated evening look.

As much of a crowning glory as long hair can be, there is nothing worse than seeing a sheaf of it completely out of condition from the shoulders down. It looks unhealthy, uncared-for and totally unbecoming. If you have long locks or are really determined to grow them, you have to realize that they require more time, enthusiasm and consideration than shorter heads of hair. The best way to make sure that your hair grows into one of those head-turning, party-stopping manes is to get into good grooming habits at an early stage.

Long hair needs to be scrutinized by a hairdresser's eagle eye just as carefully, if less frequently, than does short hair. Regular trims are still important to keep split ends at bay, although rather than attend at four to six weekly intervals, have your hair trimmed every eight to twelve weeks, depending on its condition and how quickly it seems to grow.

It is a sad fact of life that hair does grow more quickly on some women than on others and, if your hair seems to have a slow growth rate, there is nothing you can do about it, except be patient and come to terms with the fact that it

will probably never be long enough to sit on. Once your hair has grown to its full length, there is nothing you can do to make it longer. Hair grows about half an inch a month and scalp hairs usually grow for two to six years. After a scalp hair stops growing, it goes into a resting phase lasting several months before it falls out and a new hair grows. It's the length of your growing phase which determines what final length your hair will reach, and this is in your genetic make-up.

You can tell if your hair is still growing by checking the ends. The tips of normally growing, undamaged and uncut hair come to very fine points. If the ends of your hair are sharply cut, blunt or jagged, your hair is not growing to its normal length. The culprits could be all the things we have heard about before — excessive brushing with nylon brushes, excessive heat, and over-use or misuse of chemical treatments.

Even if you are growing your hair from a very short length, be sure to treat it with the kindness it deserves. Shampoo as often as necessary but make certain the product is right. You may need a different shampoo for the ends

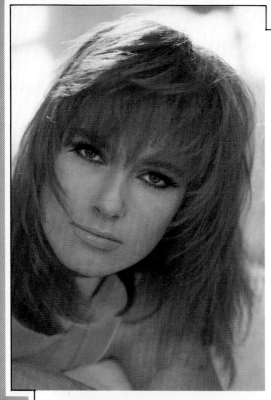

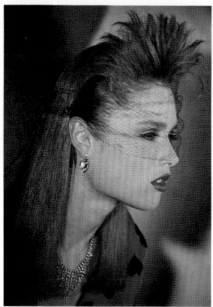

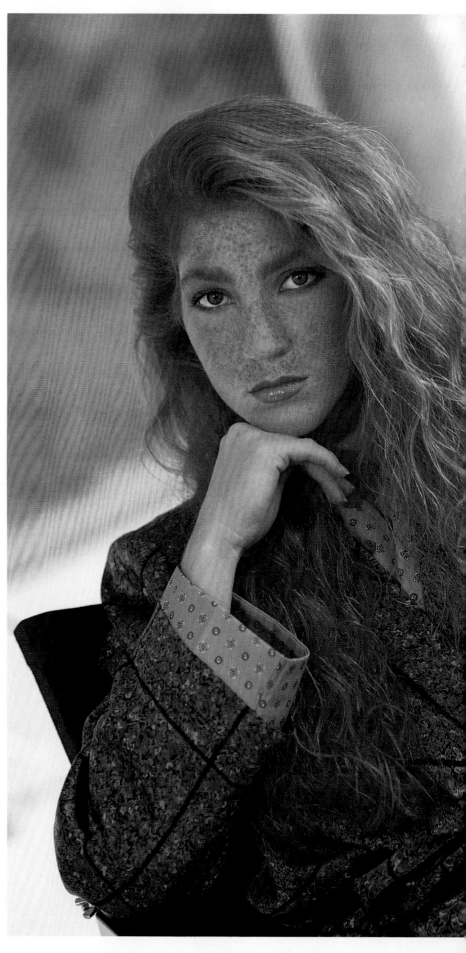

You need never get fed up with long hair, but you need patience in order to master how to style it, and time and energy to keep it in good shape. **Top:** A chic yet manageable long hair style from L'Oréal. **Above:** The front sections of this long, straight style were moussed to defy gravity and add interest (picture courtesy of Schwarzkopf). **Main picture:** Subtle highlights can do a lot to enhance long hair which might otherwise present a solid block of colour (picture courtesy of L'Oréal). **Opposite top:** Thick, wavy hair is pinned up for a loosely tousled effect. **Opposite bottom:** A few simple clips are often all that is needed to transform long straight hair into an evening style (both pictures courtesy of Schwarzkopf).

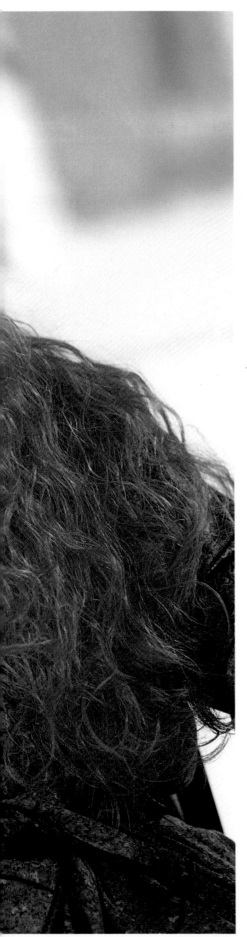
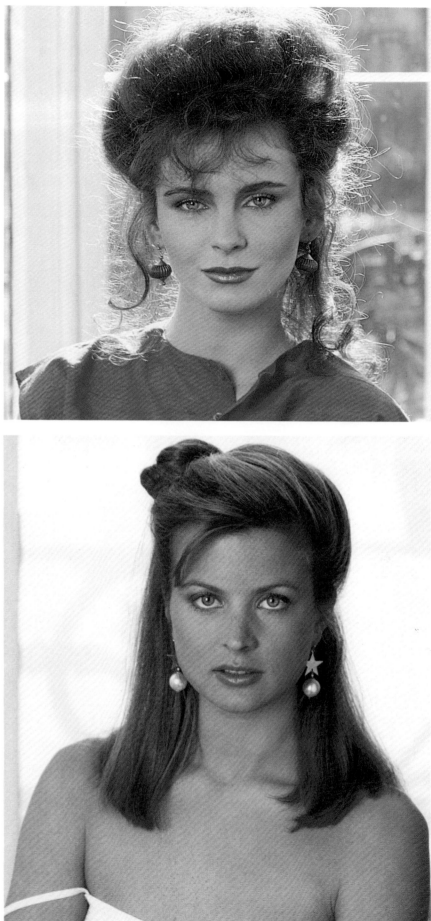

from that used for the scalp, since it is the ends which are older and require more gentle treatment. After every wash use a conditioner. This will help to smooth out the hair and make it more manageable, particularly on the mid-lengths to tips, which can become dry as they grow, or may even contain the last vestiges of a perm. In addition, use a deep, intensive conditioning treatment at least once a month. Rarely brush the hair and, when you do, use a pure bristle brush. Flip your head over and brush towards your waist. If you brush from the hairline back it can cause the hair to break. As often as possible, and particularly when the hair is wet, use a wide-toothed comb and comb in sections from the ends, so that tangles aren't dragged through from the roots. Where circumstances allow, let your hair

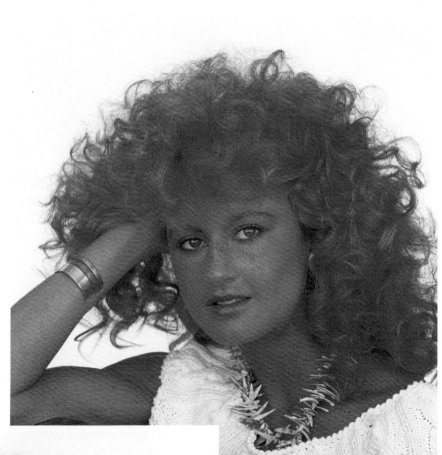

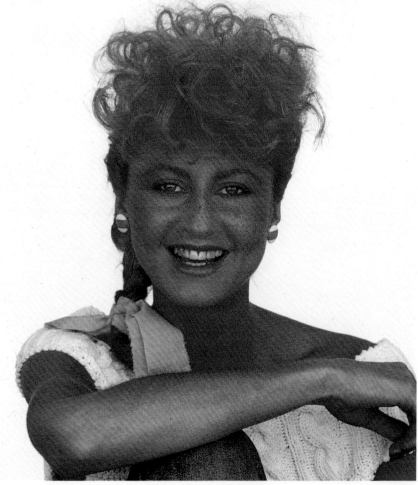

Above and left: Schwarzkopf show how this stunning curly red hair can be transformed into a cooler, sporty style for the summer months just by plaiting.

dry naturally. Blow-drying does tend to take away the natural moisture in your hair which it particularly needs when it is long. Watch your diet too. Make sure you are eating enough protein – found in lean meats, milk, cheese and eggs – as well as vitamin B – leafy green vegetables, wholemeal bread and brewer's yeast tablets.

Avoid any hairstyles which will cause the hair to be tightly pulled. It may be quick and convenient to stuff your hair in an elastic band but this could cause traction alopecia (see pp. 26–27). Instead, use covered bands and combs. Also avoid backcombing and hairspray, which could have damaging effects.

All these wise words of warning may sound terribly negative, and may leave you wondering what on earth is the point of having long hair if there are all these rules to abide by. The answer lies in versatility. There are numerous ways of styling long hair and the best person to learn from is your hairdresser. Make sure you go to someone who sympathizes with long-haired clients. If you feel your current stylist chops off too much at once, or you don't feel happy with the salon, then change. It's no good crying over lost locks when they are lying on the floor!

Look for a salon which seems geared towards long hair. A good way of telling these is by looking at the clients coming out and at the stylists themselves. If there is at least one hairdresser in the salon with long, spectacular-looking hair, it's because that salon wants to attract your custom.

Hairdressers are used to their clients wanting to grow out their hair, and now is the time for the two of you to really stick together. If you don't achieve your desire to go for growth at least once in your life then you will always regret it. Make sure that when you weaken and go grovelling into the salon pleading to have the lot off, and you will, that your stylist is firm enough to say no. That moment of despair, when you feel you cannot cope with it any longer, will be more than made up for in a few months. For this reason, it's a good idea for you and your hairdresser to work towards growth with a style in mind. That way you will have a more definite goal to achieve.

If you are growing out your hair, try to keep at least one point of interest, perhaps a fringe, rather than grow it all at once. Your hair will look tidier and still have some kind of structure to it. If your hair is already long, then, whenever you go to the salon for a trim or conditioning treatment, get your stylist to dress it in a different way so that you can take

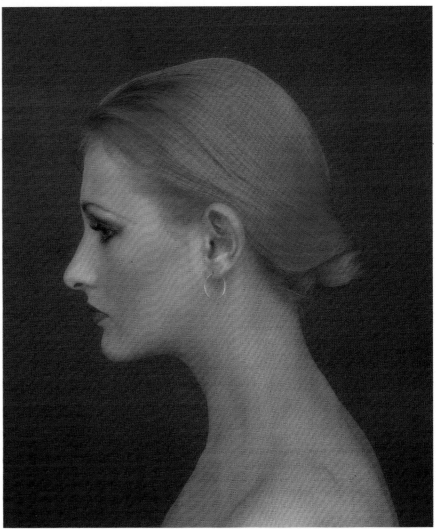

Above: Long hair never goes out of fashion — as long as you know how to update it. Christine at the Mane Line Hairdressing Salon in London swept this long head of hair back into a smooth basic chignon style.

the idea home, adapt it and eventually do it yourself.

For even more versatility, temporary waves in long straight hair can be achieved by using the colourful bendy rollers available. They can be used on dry hair for a quick lift, or on damp hair for plenty of movement. They are also comfortable to sleep in if you want to create a mane of tumbling curls the next morning.

As an alternative to a traditional plait, try twisting your hair instead. First, draw the hair back into a ponytail high on the head, and then section the ponytail into two. Next twist each section to the right, while crossing them right over left to get the main twist. Secure the twist with

coloured ribbons to finish off. Simple scarves and ribbons can be an easy and inexpensive way of jazzing up long hair. Try brushing the hair upside down and *slightly* backcombing to give maximum fullness. Once the body is there, tie a scarf around the head and matching or contrasting ribbons around the mid-sections of the hair. For a dressier, more fun look for the evening, brush the hair back off the face and tie it into a ponytail. Twist the ponytail and wrap it into a very tight chignon. Secure it with grips and decorate.

Patience is an essential virtue with long hair but, with a little time and effort on your part, you can soon build up a wardrobe of lovely long hair looks.

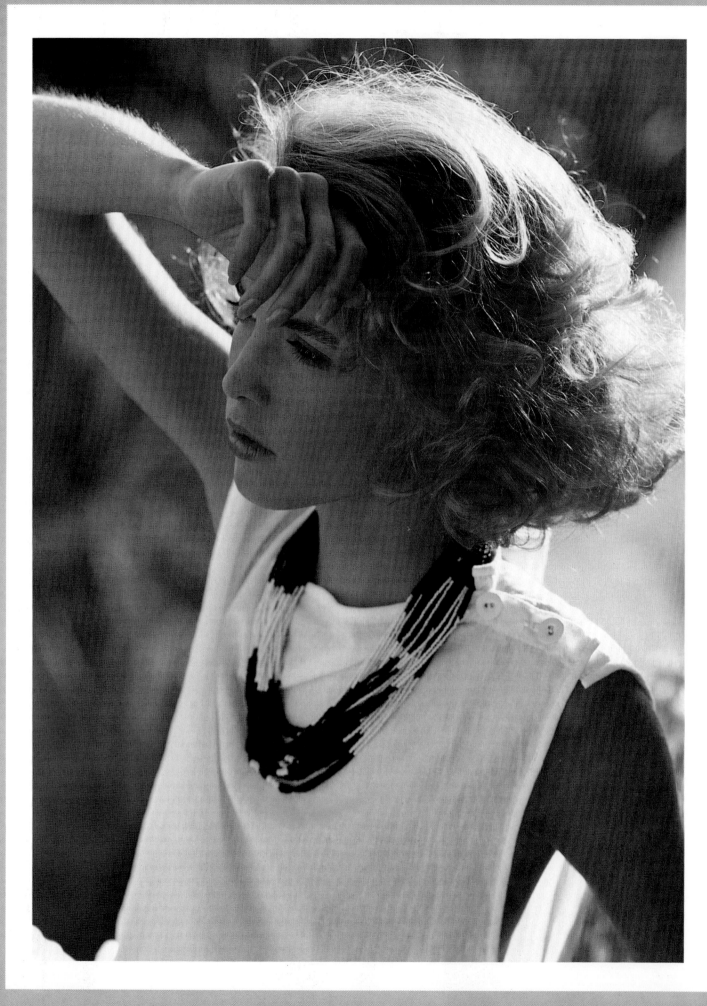

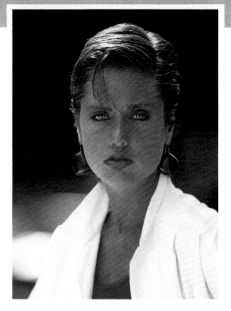

Shine on

When we wash our softest woollen sweaters, we handle them with care and use fabric conditioner. Our bodies are bathed and moisturized with soothing oils and lotions. But our hair we abuse and misuse until it does the only thing it can – it becomes dry, brittle and eventually breaks. We already know that to really get the best out of our hair we have to put the best in; that to treat it with courtesy and common sense while it is still living – underneath the scalp – will achieve the best results when it actually becomes visible. We can enhance these good locks, and to some degree improve the appearance of damaged ones, by habitually using a conditioner. After-shampoo conditioners work on the surface, or outer layer, of the hair shaft (or cuticle) and are mildly acidic. Because of their acidity they close the cuticle, which has become raised and damaged through wear and tear,

and coat the hair shaft, giving it the appearance of health and vitality. Whether or not your hair is exceptionally damaged, it is always a good idea to use a more intensive conditioner – a restructurant or protein pack – on a regular basis. Before we look more closely at this kind of conditioning treatment, let's go over what causes hair damage and thus makes the use of conditioners necessary.

Physical damage to hair may be caused by natural elements such as sunlight, drying winds, or water with a high mineral content. Daily swimming in a chlorinated pool is lethal where hair is concerned because it dries out. Damage can also be caused unnaturally from over-use of appliances such as heated rollers, which have points that can split and break the hair and damage the scalp. Hot tongs and brushes can burn and singe the hair. Incorrect backcombing and brushing can cause it to break. Added to the fact that hair can be chemically damaged by improper use of perming and colouring, it may seem that you are fighting a losing battle from the outset; you are not. If that were true we should all be going around with

hair that resembles nothing more than soggy straw!

Dry hair may also be unmanageable and difficult to comb. Manageability is affected by the overall condition of the hair, which takes into account porosity, elasticity, texture, and appearance. When one of these natural qualities is lost or weakened the hair is damaged. But let us look at each quality in turn to see precisely what they mean.

Porosity of the hair refers to the amount of liquid a strand can absorb. Damaged hair is said to be over-porous if the imbricated outer layers of the cuticle are in an open position.

Elasticity is the degree to which a hair can be stretched without breaking. This also relates to its tensile strength. A hair can be stretched almost 50% when wet, but only 10–20% when dry. If the hair is damaged, it will be very weak and break easily when stretched. The feel and diameter of the hair shaft are its texture. If the hair shaft feels smooth, hard and glossy then the imbricated outer layers are lying flat against the hair shaft and all is well. When the hair is damaged the imbrications are open and the hair feels rough. Damaged hair is dull and its appearance lacks any kind of sheen.

To help rectify all this, protein treatments actually penetrate through the cuticle into the cortex where they form temporary bonds which help to strengthen the hair and improve its texture. The size of the molecules which form the protein helps to determine how well a conditioner will work on the hair, and the best proteins are very small – small enough to penetrate the hair's cuticle layer and to adhere to the damaged part. Despite all this, do remember that intensive conditioning treatments are not magic wands. One treatment and your problem will not vanish; you will probably need a series of them to notice a real improvement. If your hair is in fairly good condition it's a sensible idea to use one every three to four weeks, as prevention is always better than cure. If your hair is badly damaged, then you may need a treatment once a week.

If your hair has really suffered in the name of fashion, or you are worried about it, it will be money well invested if you visit a trichologist, someone who has made it their profession to study the science of hair and hair care. Watch for the initials MIT or AIT at any trichological practice. This means that the practitioner is a Member of the Institute of Trichologists, or an Associated Member who has completed a minimum of three years' paramedical study, and who has passed all the exams conducted by the Institute under the supervision of qualified medical practitioners and scientists. Trichologists used to be ageing gentlemen in white coats, and a visit to one was only considered in cases of dire emergency. Nowadays trichologists are getting younger and more progressive all the time, and their clients often visit them for preventative or cosmetic reasons rather than for cures. During a

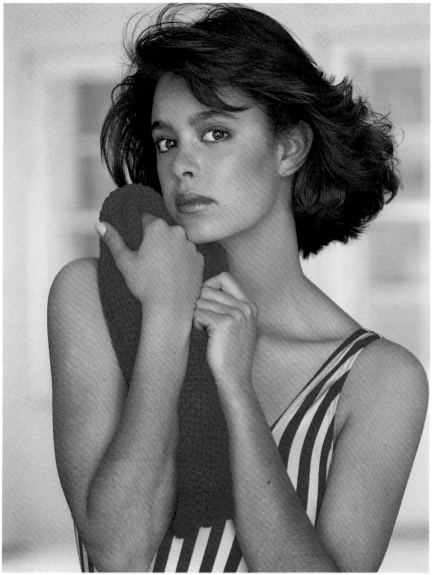

Healthy shiny hair is the result of the hair shaft's outer layers lying flat, giving it a glossy look (picture courtesy of L'Oréal).

consultation, the trichologist will examine your hair and scalp closely and may take hair samples to test. He will ask questions about your general health, your diet and what you do to your hair, and he may even look at your family history. In most cases he will be able to make an immediate diagnosis and be able to prescribe treatment and medication then and there.

If a visit to a trichologist seems too drastic a step to take to keep your hair looking good – it isn't, but from about £15 upwards for an initial consultation it can be costly – you can get yourself into good habits at home just by raiding the larder. Try these treatments every three weeks:

Hot Oil Treatment for Brittle Hair: Warm two tablespoons of olive oil, and massage it into your scalp. Wring out a towel in hot water and wind it turban-style around your head. As the towel cools, wring it out again in hot water and put it back on your head. Repeat this two or three times and then shampoo and rinse your hair in the usual way.

For Moisturizing a Dry Scalp: Beat together one egg, one tablespoon of vinegar and two tablespoons of vegetable oil just before you are ready to use it. Massage the mixture well into your scalp and comb through your hair. Leave for 15 minutes before shampooing and rinsing well.

Protein Treatment for All Hair Types: Beat two eggs together and slowly add one tablespoon of olive oil, one tablespoon of glycerine and one teaspoon of cider vinegar. Apply this after you have shampooed and rinsed once. Leave the mixture on your scalp for 15–30 minutes and then rinse off well.

Summer hair care

Whether you have an outside job which leaves you exposed to hot summer days or are about to embark on an exotic island holiday, making sure your hair is kept in peak condition and is not over-exposed to the damaging elements of sun, sea and sand are more important than ever. A holiday can make you feel on top of the world but can be your hair's deadliest enemy.

The easiest way of preventing any damage to your hair from the sun is to fend off its harmful rays by wearing a wide-brimmed hat or headscarf. However, this may not be practical and can be uncomfortable when the heat is really intense. It's a good idea to rinse your hair thoroughly after swimming but, if you are the kind who plunges in for a quick cooling dip every 20 or 30 minutes and you are on a remote beach, you are either going to be walking constantly from the shower to the sea or the facilities simply will not be available. The easiest way of protecting your hair in these conditions is to slick it back with gel, conditioner or a specially formulated hair protector. All you have to do is comb the product through your hair so that it acts as a barrier between the hair and the sun. Remember that, just like suntan lotion, you will need to apply the product again after every swim. You will have to shampoo and rinse it out thoroughly every evening, but the chances are that on holiday you will be washing your hair daily anyway.

Do try to avoid any chemical treatments a good few weeks before you go on holiday. The sun will play havoc with permed hair and give it the frizzies, and coloured hair will fade in direct sunlight – sometimes quite

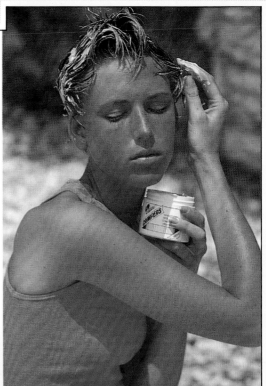

Right: A coating of conditioner can protect hair from the damaging rays of the sun (picture courtesy of the Crimpers Hair Salons in London).
Below: Summer hair care pays dividends with stunning looks like this one from L'Oréal.

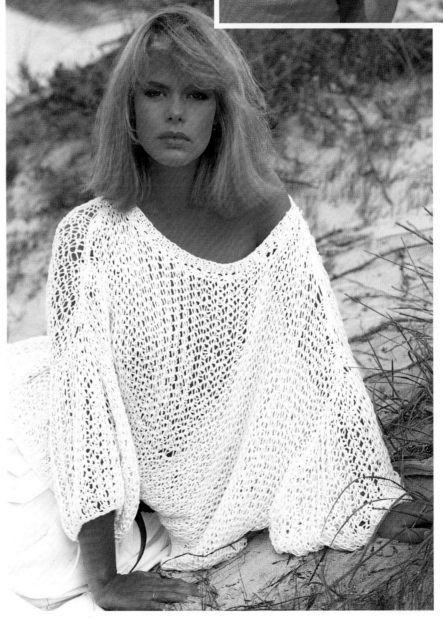

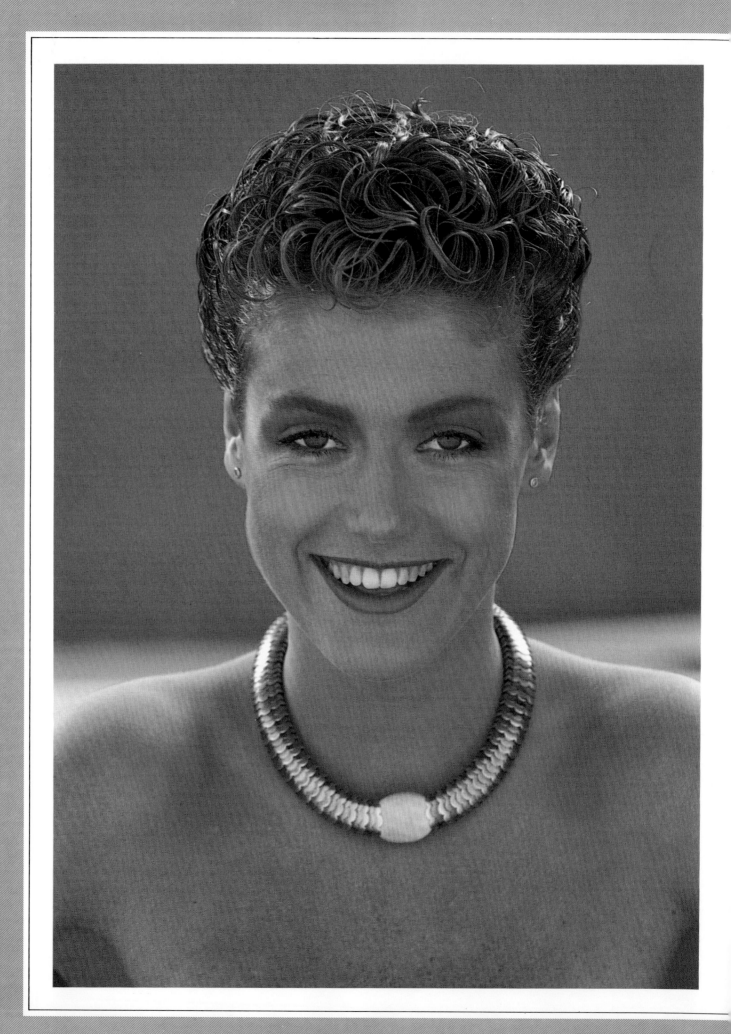

dramatically. There is no doubt that a short sharp cut a week or so before you go away is the easiest method of handling holiday hair. But don't despair; if you really don't want to have your hair cut there are ways and means of handling it!

After you have slicked back your hair, tuck a comb into one side with a bow or flower attached to it. You will look like a real bird of paradise! For getting hair neatly off your face while you are sightseeing or shopping, apply a little mousse to give it body and then tie a long strip of lace around your hair, ending up with a bow on top or on the side. Tease hair around the lace for a softening effect. You can keep hair back off your face, or brighten it up once it has been gelled back, by tying around it a thick plait made with colourful skeins of wool. Long hair can be firmly gelled back, folded under in a twist, and secured in place with a covered band and bow clip. Wrap some prettily patterned cotton voile once around the back of the head and tie the ends into a loose knot on the crown for a blaze of colour. Don't forget that, no matter how unattractive your hair feels when it has been slicked back, it can look cool, cute and chic when accompanied by a low-necked vest and shorts for lunch-time snacks or tea-time chats.

A little bit of attention goes a long way when it comes to holidays, and what better way to enhance that tan when you get home than with a gleaming, healthy head of hair.

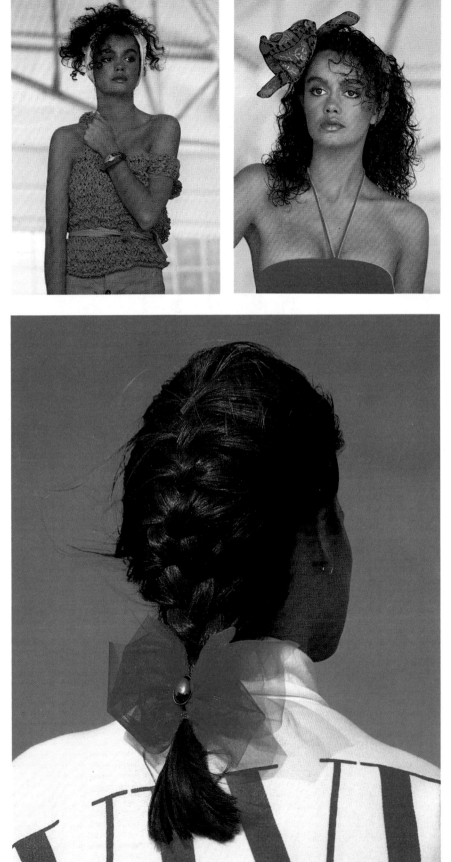

Left: Protecting your hair from harsh sunlight doesn't necessarily mean that you have to look, and feel, unglamorous as this style from L'Oréal shows. **Top, left and right:** These hair styles, also from L'Oréal, show how different hair can look with the help of simple accessories such as ribbons and bands. **Right:** A neat plait is tied with a bright scarf for extra holiday dazzle (picture courtesy of L'Oréal).

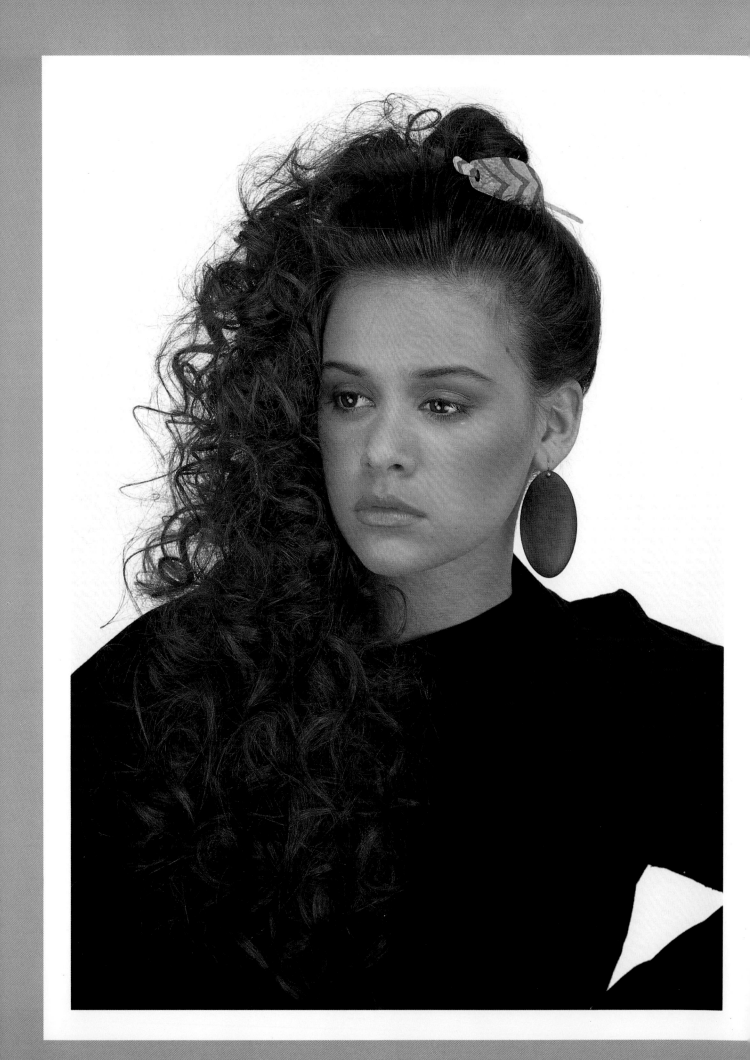

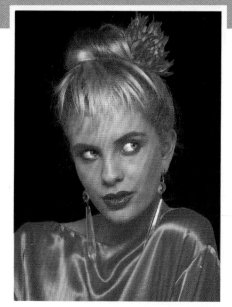

Hair accessories

The choice has never been so wide, the colour schemes never so vibrant. Whatever your passion – ribbons, clips, scarves, slides or combs – hair accessories are there in abundance. They are fun to use, are often a practical way of keeping the hair tidy while it is growing, and can be a valuable accessory to any outfit.

When selecting your hair accessories, beware of falling into the 'cheap and cheerful' trap. Inexpensive, flimsy slides and combs may look lovely on the display stand but, in practice, may be totally incapable of holding your hair for any length of time. It's always worth consulting your hairdresser before you actually buy a hair accessory. He or she will be able to tell you which would best suit your hair type and style and, if they are particularly keen to help you grow your hair, will be eager to show you how to make the best use of them. It's even worth paying out a few extra

Opposite: One of a wide choice of hair accessories to hold these long curly locks high on the head. **Above:** Floral garlands were among the three most popular forms of primitive hairdressing (pictures courtesy of the Molton Brown Hair Salon, London).

pounds on a wash in the salon so that the stylist can then explain and demonstrate how to put them in – many a good hair accessory has fallen by the wayside because of its owner's sheer inability to get to grips with it.

Hair accessories and ornaments may be brighter and more beautiful than ever before, but they are certainly not new. The earliest forms of hair ornament were used among the primitive races who adopted three chief methods of hairdressing: the floral garland, plaits intermingled with strings of shells, and hair dressed with a fatty substance and held in place with a wooden pin or comb. Sound familiar? Between these primitive designs and modern styles there are a wealth of ornamental head-dresses which flourished during early civilizations, and many of them can still be seen in national museums. Ancient Egyptian women wore their hair at shoulder length in numerous fine plaits, decorated with coloured silk. For state occasions crown-like ornaments replaced silk, and these often took the form of a bird designed as if perched on the head, with its wings covering the hair on either side. In contrast Greek

women around 500 B.C. often tied their hair up in a knot, securing it with a single valuable pin,

Some Arab tribes wore their hair braided with tiny pieces of coral or miniature metal bells, whereas Greeks and Romans were very fond of mounting pearls on a flat cap on a little bar of gold. A series of tiny discs, like little coins, one above the other at the end of the shaft of a pin, was a popular form of hair decoration in about 600 B.C. Hairpins were also ornate, and early bronze specimens in England dating from before the Roman invasion display elegance and originality.

Before Christianity was introduced the druidesses would place wreaths of verbena, considered a sacred plant, on their heads prior to visiting the temple altars.

For a long time during the Middle Ages women's hair ornaments were all based on the idea of the crown. Unmarried women wore rose crowns, and the cultivation of rose gardens and the art of making such crowns ranked high among women's occupations. They did not entirely replace the brooch or comb, however, which from Saxon times onwards were

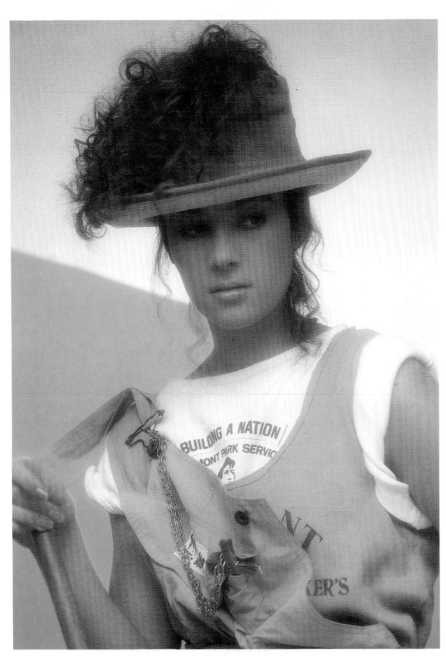

If you've got to get ahead, get a hat! This picture from *Hair & Beauty* magazine shows how even hats can be adapted to accessorize longer styles.

piled her locks on top of her head and secured them with a garter ribbon! Although the garter ribbon didn't quite become the mode, Spanish combs were introduced to hold the curls in place. Some of the styles based on this were extremely elaborate and are still being copied and used today. Later in the 18th century huge headdresses were introduced, topped by great turbans and decorated with swaying feathers. In England feathers were the favourite hair ornament. Ostrich and heron feathers were dyed myriad colours – yellow, black, blue, green, lilac, gold and silver. Even for mourning, gauze bonnets were worn, perched on the curls, with a white and black feather gracing the look. Tortoise-shell and enamel were favoured materials for Spanish and side combs, and some of the most lovely of these were used to complete hairstyles by famous hairdressers of the Second Empire in Paris in 1860–70. Parisian hairdressers at this time employed skilled designers to make combs for their clientele. Favourite types of side comb of the period were blond or brown tortoise-shell mounted with golden balls. Some of these classic styles have proved so popular, and have such everlasting quality and appeal, that they are still being imitated today.

At the beginning of the 20th century, the long hairstyles fashionable at the time were piled on top of the head and pads or false hair were added to give increased bulk. In 1908 the innovative young designer Paul Poiret helped to popularize the fashion of wearing scarves and turbans around the hair, using materials and colours that complemented the dress. For evening wear, oriental-type turbans were often worn, and these were decorated at the front with feathers or a cluster of jewels.

After the First World War, long hairstyles were often pinned up near the crown and held in place with an ornate comb, a band

the most usual forms of hair ornaments.

In the medieval period a tall dunce-like cap called the hennin, covered in silk and carrying a floating veil, was introduced into England from France. Older women sometimes wore a divided hennin, giving the effect of a star or horned headdress. These were followed by the Juliet styles – where hair would be divided into two long plaits adorned with a small jewelled or embroidered cap.

A hair ornament of a different kind was *la ferronière*, a jewel worn high in the middle of the forehead which was kept in place by a fine gold chain around the head. It was introduced by a favourite of Francis I, king of France. There have been many variations on this style of ornament which lends itself to an otherwise simple hairstyle.

The fontange, or high coiffure, of the Queen Anne period was named after a duchess who, having lost her hairpins while hunting, or scarf often being worn round the head for evening wear. Then the world of hair fashion was revolutionized by the new short hairstyles, and these paved the way for the helmet-like cloche hats which were pulled down right to the eyebrows and covered all the hair except for a small curl or wave forward on the cheeks. Once hair became longer again the cloche hats were not suitable and went out of favour.

During World War II, when many women were working in factories, hair had to be covered with a scarf to prevent it getting caught in machinery, and this style was often worn in leisure time as well, particularly by older women. Other wartime styles returned to using combs to pin the hair on top of the head, or a band was put on the crown and the hair was swept over it to form a continuous roll right round the head, this method of dressing being called a Victory Roll.

The 1950s saw long hair being tied back into a ponytail springing from the crown of the head, and the swinging ponytail was a very characteristic feature of the decade. This loose style was superseded in the early 1960s by the contrived backcombed beehives, which were often crowned with curls or false hair. Later in the swinging sixties, coincident with the hippy and flower-power movements, hairstyles became much freer and girls often wore flowers in their hair.

When the extraordinary punk styles of the second half of the 1970s had burnt themselves out as high fashion, more natural styles became popular again and now hair is often held or tied back with coloured scarves or bands, particularly by sporty women.

In the early 1980s a method of dressing hair — for it's much more than an accessory — took London by storm and is now ready to take hair design well into the 21st century. Hair extensions were the brainchild of an innovative London hairdresser, Simon Forbes, who realized how inhibiting and frustrating the natural growth rate of hair — half an inch per month — could be. His hair extensions are achieved by weaving specially formulated mono-fibre strands into the natural hair and heat-sealing them. Almost any colour effect can be achieved with hair extensions, which last for about four months and can be washed as normal hair would be during this time. They can be styled to look as pretty or as punk as your own individual style dictates and if, after four months, you don't want them any more your hair has grown a tidy two inches! Ask your hairdresser about hair extensions. He should be able to obtain them and put them in for you or know where you can get them. They have lasting quality and are certainly a painless way of growing out an old style. Study the pictures of the more popular hair accessory ideas, and remember that practice makes perfect.

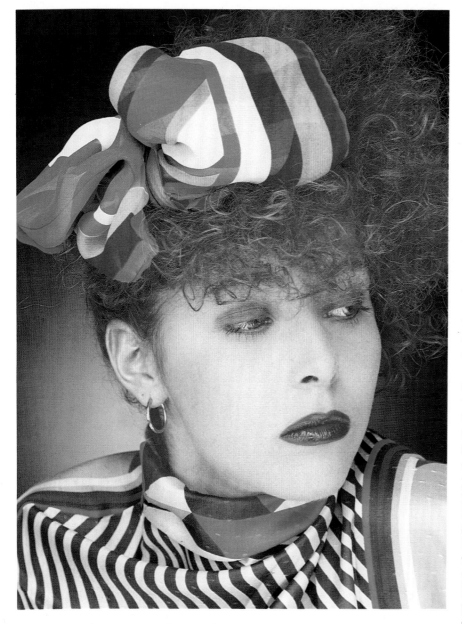

Scarves have been worn to decorate hair since time immemorial. In this picture, Christine from the Mane Line Hair Salon in London has brushed the hair up from the nape and pinned it with a silk bow, allowing the curls to spiral forward on to the brow.

Below: A style of pure fantasy heavily accessorized by London hairdresser John Dacosta. **Right:** *Hair & Beauty* magazine show how a piece of black netting, made to act as a hat, can add subtle sophistication for the evening. **Below (main picture):** The Molton Brown Hair Salon in London have used their dayglow hairknots to achieve a vibrant effect. **Opposite:** Christine of the Mane Line Salon in London used a simple chiffon scarf to decorate and tidy this long, tousled look.

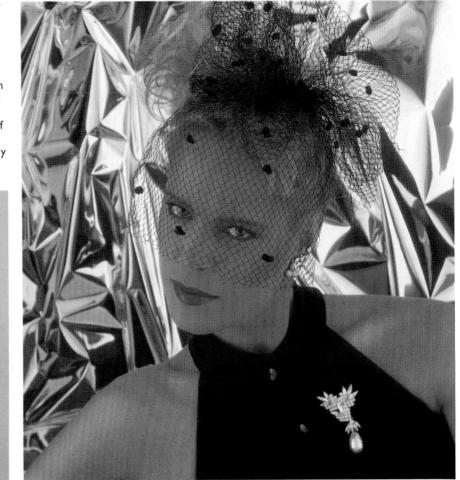

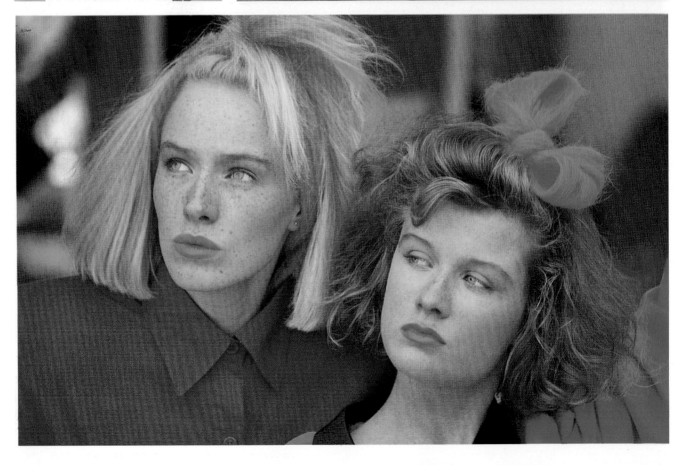

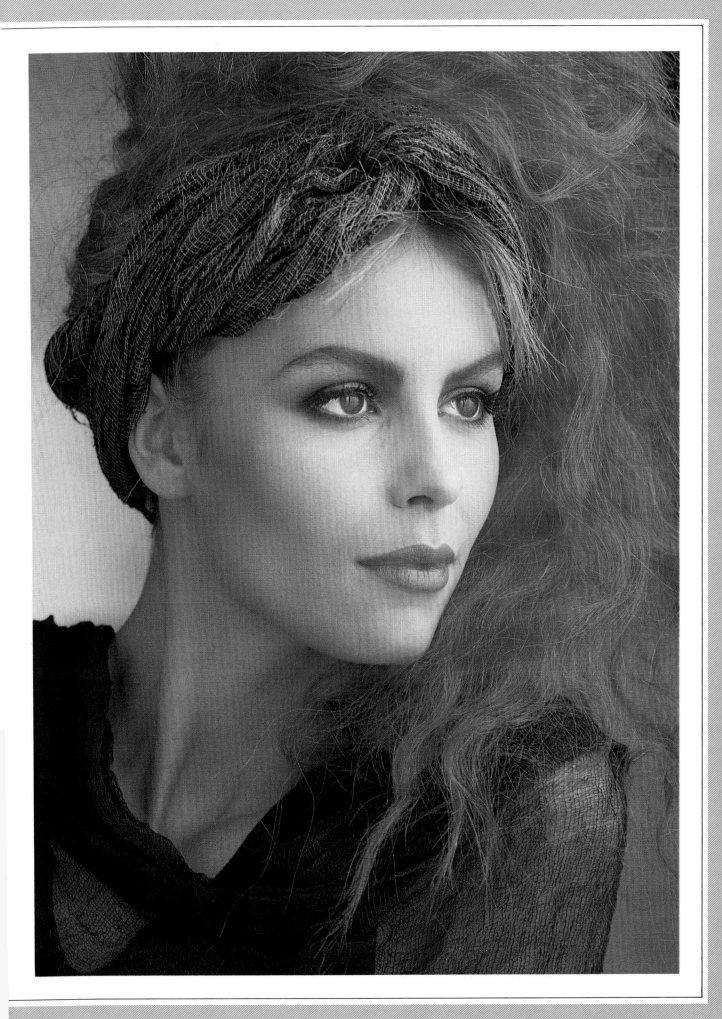

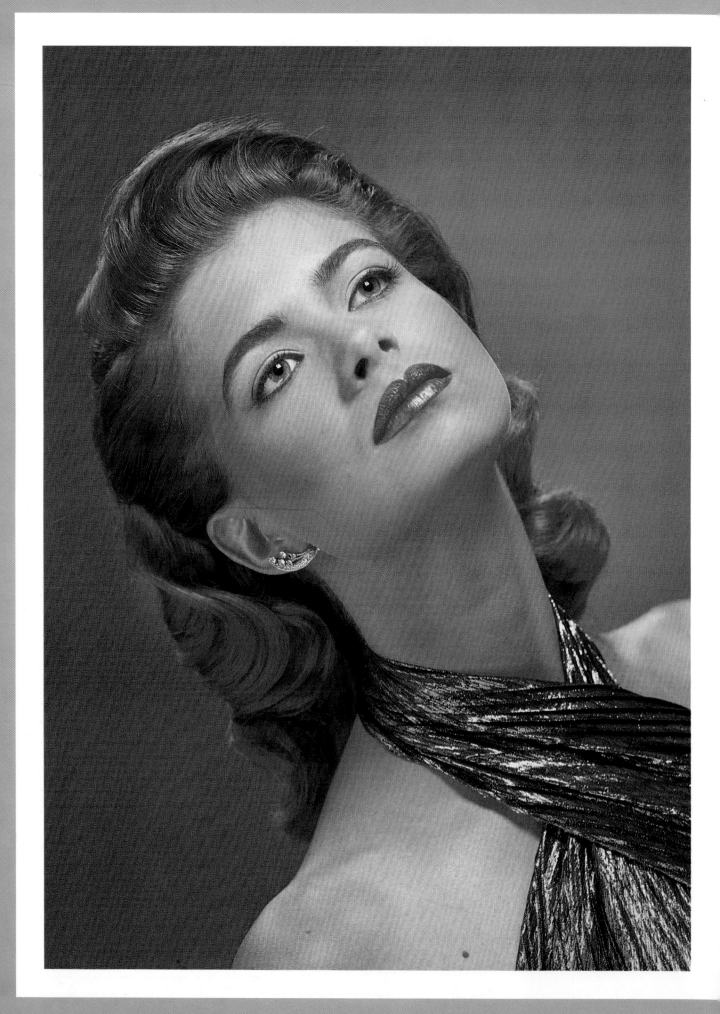

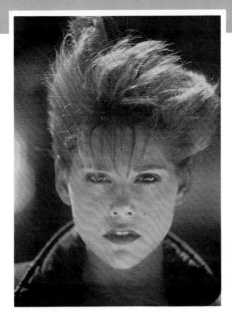

A history of hairstyles

Techniques may become more and more progressive and styles increasingly avant-garde, but hairdressing is a craft which has been with us since the beginnings of civilization. In some cases fashions didn't change very much for hundreds of years, and trends in hair design would overlap and repeat themselves as much as fashion does today. Athens once set the fashion for the ancient world, and around 500 B.C. Greek women would wear their hair knotted on the crown and held by a pin or in loose tresses around the shoulders.

From about 100 B.C. to about A.D. 100 Egyptian women wore their hair in thin plaits with fringes on the forehead. These plaits were sometimes fastened together in twos or threes at the ends.

The Romans brought their hairstyles to Britain from about A.D. 100 onwards but Saxon women, however, had other ideas.

They preferred single or double plaits, sometimes looped under a crown. Younger, unmarried women wore their hair in a bandeau, but otherwise loose on their shoulders. Married women did not cut their hair and in France hair was of symbolic importance, being the mark of royalty, and to cut a woman's hair was to inflict mortal injury.

The medieval period saw a number of striking hair styles. Nets were placed over the head and hair stuffed into them to form a large puff on either side. The nets were at first made of horsehair, but in time gold nets became more popular and were often topped by a turban. The hennin was later introduced from France.

During Tudor times, however, there was no attempt to use any art in dressing hair, which was allowed to fall on the shoulders from under a hood with rectangular lines. This was worn over a wimple which hid the ears and outlined the face. The French word for this Tudor hood, *chaperon*, now means a guardian for young women.

This kind of severity disappeared during Elizabethan and Stuart times when hairdressers were really called upon to display their skills – particularly wig-makers, who were kept busy by women of the court of Queen Elizabeth. Elizabeth I wore many different wigs, decorated with a variety of jewels. The manner of arranging the hair with a point on the forehead became a feature of this period, but this style was completely discarded with the arrival in England of Charles I's queen, Henrietta Maria, who came from Paris and instantly created a new trend. Her style of hairdressing, with bunches of curls on the forehead and at the side of the head, marks the Stuart era. The formal arrangements typical of the Elizabethan and Stuart eras came to an end at the close of the 17th century. First, hair was curled all over the head, then a taller style of hairdressing was introduced, called the fontange (see 'Hair accessories') in which the hair was piled on top of the head and retained by a Spanish comb.

The 18th century saw a complete about-turn. Hair tended to be dressed low and little lace bonnets became popular. Short and tightly curled hair became fashionable and this style eventually had a powdered wig modelled on it.

Having come down, the only way for powdered hairstyles to go was up, and towards the close of the 18th century women's hairstyles were so tall that ladies had to sit on the floors of coaches in order to fit in them!

At the beginning of the 19th century wigs were abandoned and there was a tendency towards styles based on wig designs. This was because it was thought too extreme to change from the voluminous wigs to natural hair, and so styles were produced to bridge that gap. As one might imagine, this led to some pretty extraordinary ways of dressing hair, a typical example of which was 'dog hairdressing'. Hair would be parted in the middle and arranged to show a thick fringe on the forehead, and then allowed to

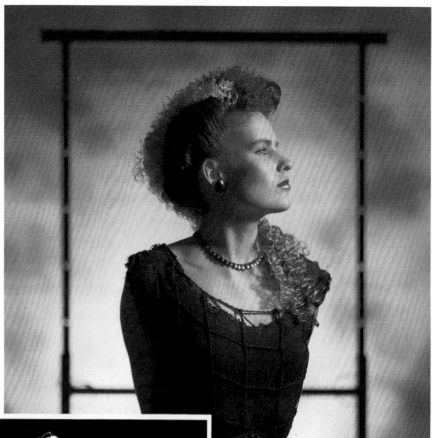

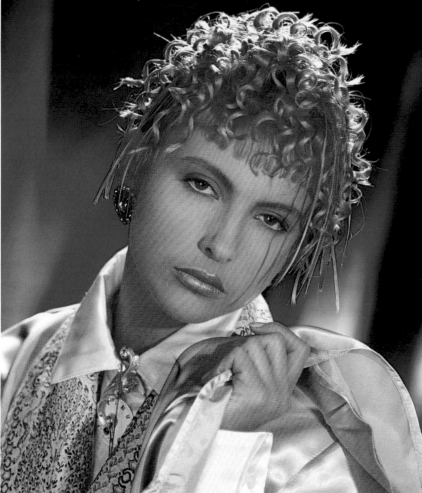

Above: A hairdressing aid of the future, hair extensions, were used to create this romantic, almost historical, head of curls by stylist John Dacosta.
Left: Ringlets are taken into the future by the Stevie Buckle Hair Salon, London.

fall on to the shoulders. It had the effect of making the wearer's head look something like a Charles II spaniel!

A more attractive hairstyle of this period was achieved by knotting the hair back off the forehead to end in a cascade of curls at the nape of the neck which would be held in place by a large comb, placed low at the back of the head.

In another popular style at the start of Queen Victoria's reign the hair was turned under at the back rather than curled. Bleaching and dyeing came into favour at this time and began to influence hairstyles, which showed much more originality. Ladies' hairdressing salons became more general and women got used to the idea of visiting them, rather than depending on the hairdressing services of their own maids.

The growth in hairdressing at this time can be to some extent attributed to the great painters of the day, who recognized a woman's hair as her chief beauty and took great pains to encourage hairdressers to dress it suitably. By the time Queen Victoria died at the beginning of the 20th century, women had their hair long and wore it piled on top of the head. As the First World War approached, styles became simpler, although the hair was still long and extended at least to the shoulders when let down.

Then came the bombshell: with the emancipation of women and the feeling that women were the equals of men, there was a general trend towards much shorter hair, and once the new bob had become accepted, it was shortened into bare-necked styles, often shaped to a point on the cheeks. An extreme example of short hair was the Eton crop, which was cut around the ears. At the end of the 1920s these shorter styles began to lose favour, and in the years leading up to the Second World War longer hair gained ground once again. Women began to dye their hair in imitation of the film stars who had risen to prominence in the early 1930s with the coming of the talkies, and blond hair became eagerly sought-after despite its artificial appearance. The late 1930s saw the introduction of long bobs, which were similar to a long page-boy style, and hair was also piled on top of the head in a variety of styles.

With the outbreak of World War II, women in the forces had to keep their hair neat and off uniform collars, although it was often still long and was simply pinned up to comply with regulations. Once the conflict had ended and fashion re-emerged,

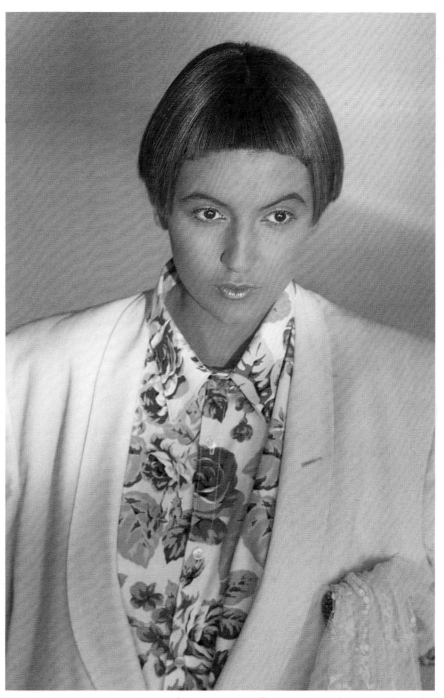

The bob is among the classics of hair creations. This one, from Lawrence Falk of the Crimpers Salons in London, is a short bob with an even shorter fringe.

the long hairstyles worn since the 1930s looked over-complicated, and short hair came into vogue once more. Mostly it was parted at the side and waved or curled at the sides and back, an extreme version being the urchin cut in 1949.

In the early 1950s, hair was fashionable in both short and long styles, and later in the decade the ponytail became very popular with younger women. Between

1955 and 1958 hairstyles began to be more contrived and were higher and fuller in appearance, an example being the French pleat in which the hair was folded down the back of the crown and pinned under.

By 1960 more fashion-conscious women had adopted even higher and fuller styles, the 'blown-up' effect being used by many right through the decade. Backcombing

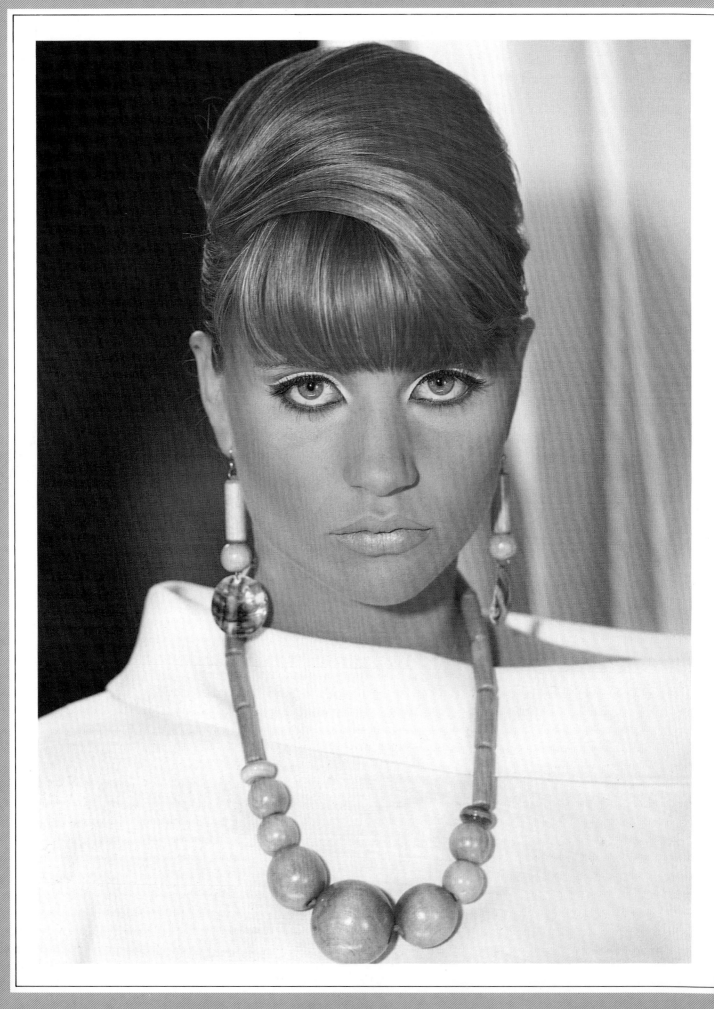

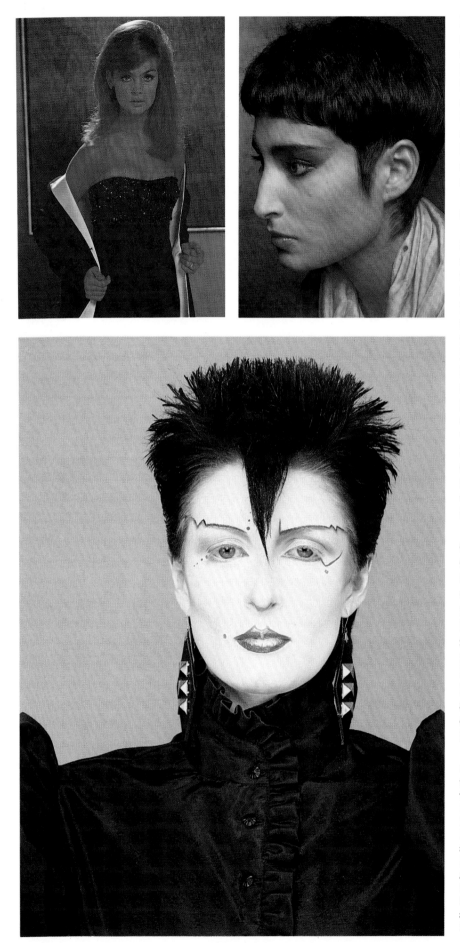

had become an everyday occurrence in hair styling, and most styles were based on a beehive or bird's-nest look. As the hippie and flower-power movements caught on after 1967, hair was grown to at least shoulder length and was common to both men and women by the early 1970s. By now high contrived styles looked very dated, and the long bobs of the 1930s and 40s came back in, giving a less set appearance.

Following the unkempt and uncared-for looks of the hippie era, women suddenly began to take much more care of their hair in the mid-1970s, and trichology became very popular. A good example of a common style was the casual, but neat and flattering look adopted by stars such as Farrah Fawcett-Majors. Then came the outrageous styles of the punk era – an expression of the attitude that 'anything goes' – with all-over spiky hair and striking colours. Soon quite extraordinary hairstyles became commonplace among younger women, with long spiky multi-coloured hair sticking out at varying angles.

However, in the 1980s these extreme styles have been toned down generally, and although hair may well still be dyed in various colours, there is a trend towards more conventional styles. If the hair is shorter it tends to be very short at the back and sides and permed on top. Women with longer hair tend to have it waved in order to make it easier to look after. More than ever, hairdressers have a great role to play in keeping women fashionable.

Opposite: It was in the late 1950s that hairstyles began to be higher and fuller than for some time before. This 1960s' recreation is from the Stevie Buckle Hair Salon, London. **Top left:** During the late 1960s hair came down again (picture courtesy of Popperfoto, London). **Top right:** Reminiscent of Ancient Egypt or a style of the future? From the Molton Brown Hair Salon in London. **Left, main picture:** An avant garde look from stylist John Dacosta.

Index

Page numbers in italics refer to illustrations

Acknowledgements

The author wishes to thank the following people and organizations who have helped with the preparation of this book: Karen Berman, Andrew Bernie, Stevie Buckle, Crimpers, John Dacosta, Christine Mitchell-Driver at Mane Line, The Taylor Ferguson Salon, Glasgow, Kate Friis, Glemby International, L'Oréal, Neutrogena, Schwarzkopf, Alberto TRESemme/Indola, Leslie Vince for the Graham Webb Salons, and Vitapointe.